FASTING FROM CANCER

Why When We Eat Might Be
Just as Important as What We Eat

Jonathan Stegall, MD

Copyright © 2023 by Jonathan Stegall, MD

All rights reserved.

No part of this book may be reproduced in any form or by any means including electronic reproduction and photocopying without written permission of the author.

ISBN : 978-1-7323273-6-8 (Print)
       978-1-7323273-8-2 (ePub)
       978-1-7323273-7-5 (Kindle)

Interior design by Booknook.biz

To my beautiful wife, Carrie. You are an amazing woman who inspires me to be a better man.

Table of Contents

Chapter 1   The Cancer Conundrum 1
Chapter 2   An Introduction to Fasting................ 27
Chapter 3   From Feasting to Fasting 45
Chapter 4   Fasting and Cancer...................... 67
Chapter 5   What About When I'm Not Fasting? 95
Chapter 6   Your Nutritional Foundation 103
Chapter 7   What to Have in Moderation.............. 125
Chapter 8   Things You Should Minimize.............. 147
Chapter 9   How to Fast 159

APPENDIX

Appendix I   What Is Integrative Oncology? 185

CHAPTER 1

The Cancer Conundrum

There are three words that no person ever wishes to hear themselves, or hear told to a loved one: "You have cancer." Yet today, women have a 1 in 3 lifetime chance of developing cancer. For men, the odds are a grim 1 in 2. (1) Cancer is poised to soon overtake heart disease as the number one killer of people in the developed world.

In the pantheon of diseases, perhaps none strike as much fear into a person's soul as cancer does. For a disease so prevalent, it often shows no symptoms, silently setting our health up for destruction until it is finally detected in later stages when treatments are more severe and prognoses grimmer. Furthermore, the fear that the pain of treatment can exceed the pain caused by the disease itself is an overwhelming feeling. This feeling is not unfounded; many of us have watched as cancer treatments have ravaged those we love. Perhaps you have experienced that agony yourself. For all of our advancements in medicine, the prospect of going through cancer remains a terrifying prospect for patients.

The above paints a bleak picture, but I want you to know that there is hope. That hope is the motivation behind this book. While cancer is a formidable adversary, we can collectively do better than we are currently doing in our fight against this disease. In fact, we *must* do better. The good news is that there is mounting evidence showing that we already have many of the tools available to both prevent cancer and treat it more effectively. The goal of this book is to empower you with knowledge gleaned from emerging research as well as what I see in my oncology practice every day. My hope is that this will assist you greatly, whether you are hoping to prevent cancer or you are currently fighting it.

Why We Must Do Better

Cancer is not necessarily a disease of modernity. The ancient Egyptians were the first to describe cancer in a papyrus scroll known as the Edwin Smith papyrus. They were also the first to document their attempts at surgical removal of cancer tumors, as cancer has even been detected in the remains of ancient Egyptian mummies. (2, 3) The ancient Greeks are also known to have recognized and categorized cancer as a disease. Hippocrates, known as the father of medicine, gave cancer its first name, *carcinos*, the Greek word for *crab*. This was likely chosen to describe the spindling tendrils emanating from cancerous tumors. (2, 4, 5) Eventually, the Romans would translate *carcinos* to *carcinoma*, nomenclature we still use today. (2) Ultimately, we know that cancer has coexisted with us as long as we have inhabited Earth.

While the presence of cancer is nothing new, what is both uniquely modern and incredibly disturbing is the alarming rate at which it afflicts people today. For the time being, cancer is second only to heart disease in terms of lives lost per year. It is rare today to find someone who has not been affected by cancer in some way.

Worldwide, cancer represents an enormous burden. In 2018, over 18 million new cases of cancer were diagnosed, and 9.6 million people were estimated to have perished as a result. This data was collected using reliable reporting methods in 185 countries out of the 195 countries total countries worldwide. Thus, these statistics likely fall short of the true burden. (6) The number of new cancer cases per year is expected to rise to over 23.6 million people by 2030, and the World Health Organization (WHO) predicts that worldwide cancer deaths will exceed 13 million people per year by then. (7, 8) With the number of cases and deaths so high, it is not unreasonable to think of cancer not just as an epidemic, but a pandemic affecting the entire world. And our experience in 2020 highlights the scale of just how burdensome cancer is.

At the time of this writing, tens of millions of people are known to have been infected with the novel coronavirus. Millions are thought to have died from COVID-19, the disease caused by the virus, over the last few years. Certainly, the reason why a novel, deadly virus has galvanized the world's medical communities to find treatments and cures is clear. But given the yearly burden of cancer—with deaths and cases eclipsing those even of a worldwide pandemic—it is unclear why these numbers have not elicited a stronger response from the world's governing bodies. While we hope the pain and suffering caused by the novel coronavirus will eventually be a footnote in history, cancer will likely remain a chronic problem that continues to worsen.

While the global numbers are staggering, cancer's burden in the United States seems to be particularly heavy. In 2023, it is expected that there will be over 1.9 million new cases of cancer diagnosed in the United States, with over 600,000 Americans dying from cancer. (9) This means that cancer cases in the US represent roughly 10% of new cancer cases diagnosed every year worldwide, even though the United States' population makes up far less than 10% of the world's population. In other words, cancer incidence in the US is unusually high. If we are honest, we must admit that cancer has been ravaging this country for quite some time.

In the 1970s, cancer rates had spiked to levels never seen before, prompting president Richard Nixon to declare war on cancer. This war allocated massive amounts of money for cancer research in search of better diagnostics, more effective treatments, and an elusive cure. Since then, there have been some incredible strides in cancer detection, diagnosis, and treatment. Cancer is not the death sentence that it once was, which affirms the fact that standards of care—including surgery, radiation, chemotherapy, and the burgeoning field of immunotherapy—are powerful tools in our fight against cancer and should not be ignored, even by those more "natural" or "alternative" minded.

Yet no matter how much better we have gotten at treating cancer, its incidence has continued to rise. The staggering rise in incidence raises some important questions. For example, are cancer rates worse than ever before, or are there other factors skewing our data, making the results seem worse or more frightening than they actually are?

Many researchers argue that the rate of cancer is increasing simply because our methods of diagnosing cancer have improved. Plus, people are generally living longer than they once did. Based on this information, we would conclude that cancer has always been this prevalent;

we're just living long enough to develop it. And when we do develop it, we are better at finding it. These are valid points, but there is research pointing toward the fact that this is an incomplete picture of cancer incidence.

A 2012 study in the *New England Journal of Medicine* sought to determine the most prevalent causes of death from 1900 to 2010. This particular study focused on the number of deaths per 100,000 people caused by specific diseases. What the researchers found was worrisome. In 1900, cancer was responsible for claiming the lives of 64 out of every 100,000 people. By the 1970s, cancer was the cause of death in 162 people out of every 100,000. By 2010, 184 deaths out of every 100,000 people were caused by cancer—more than triple the rate of 1900. (10)

Another study published in the *British Journal of Cancer* in 2015 sought to discern the increase in lifetime risk of developing cancer. The study found that a woman who was born in 1930 had a 36.7% risk of developing cancer in her lifetime. For a woman born in 1960, that risk rose to 47.5%. For men, the statistics were more grim. A man born in 1930 had a 38.5% chance of developing cancer over his lifetime. For a man born in 1960, that risk was elevated to 53.5%. Ultimately, for any person born after 1960, the risk of developing cancer was greater than 50%, representing a 1 in 2 chance. (11)

Yet another study published in the *Journal of the National Cancer Institute* found that people born after 1990 have twice the risk of developing colon cancer and quadruple the risk of developing rectal cancer. (12) These are significant increases!

Research also points toward the incidence of multiple types of cancer rising. More specifically, gastrointestinal cancers, skin cancers, liver cancer, thyroid cancer, pancreatic cancer, endometrial cancer, and cancers caused by certain viruses are all increasing. (13, 14)

It is difficult and perhaps shortsighted to blame what amounts to a global pandemic simply on better testing and slightly longer average lifespans. Ultimately, even adjusting for these two factors, the reality remains that our lifetime risk of developing cancer is virtually 1 in 2, which is higher than it has ever been. Furthermore, cancer rates in younger adults are on the rise, meaning cancer is not relegated to being called a disease of old age. There simply must be other factors involved when it comes to the incidence of cancer, and we must do more to understand these factors. Roughly 50 years after President Nixon declared war on cancer, despite the billions of dollars spent on research, people continue to be diagnosed with cancer at an alarming rate. While our methods of detecting and treating cancer have dramatically improved, it would be difficult to say—in light of the enormous burden cancer continues to place on society on both a domestic and a global scale—that we are winning the war on cancer.

Why This Book Is Necessary

In light of the above, it can be easy to think that there is little to be done to stop cancer in its tracks. Certainly, after decades, even centuries, of studying cancer, and the investment of billions (maybe even trillions) of dollars, it seems that we are no closer to a cure. Cancer and its treatments remain a scourge, and it seems that a void exists in terms of advice on how to prevent cancer.

I believe all of this is on the cusp of changing.

When I decided to become an oncologist, it was so I could make a difference in people's lives. I wanted to help people walk through a journey no one wants to make. I believed in the beginning—and I believe now—that there is much more we can (and should) be doing in our fight against cancer. This belief and commitment to helping people in my practice have led me to forge a unique path in treating cancer. The result of my conventional medical training in oncology combined with my own research into what many consider "alternative" medicine has culminated in what I call *integrative oncology*.

In my practice, we combine the best of both conventional and alternative cancer treatments. In 2018, I published a bestselling book called *Cancer Secrets*, which was an in-depth look at what integrative oncology has to offer to the greater discussion on cancer. I believe that the results I have achieved are promising, and I remain hopeful and excited about the future of integrative oncology.

Cancer Secrets is not necessarily required reading to understand the information in this book. I want people who have never heard of me, my practice, or my first book to have an idea about what we do, so we will cover some of that, because it is important to our ends in this book. One of the things I have learned is that there is much more power that lies within a patient's hands than they are often led to believe. Much of the emerging research backs this up.

Since I published *Cancer Secrets*, there has been significant scientific inquiry into the discipline of fasting. The science that has emerged leads me to believe that this very simple yet powerful tool may be one of the most important and overlooked ways to fight cancer. Simply put, it is not just what you do or do not eat that can play a role in cancer prevention and treatment. While these are important factors, we are learning that when and how much you eat might be just as important.

Before we get to fasting, however, it is important to understand a few things about what cancer is and what it is not.

What Is Cancer?

Cancer is a broad, encompassing term used to describe over 100 separate diseases, but if we are to summarize what cancer is, it is best to describe it as our own normal cells going rogue. Our bodies contain between 40 and 100 trillion cells which are the building blocks of every living organism. Cells form tissues, and tissues form organs, which perform all the functions necessary for life.

Different cells in the body perform different functions depending on what tissues they compose. For example, cells that make up the heart perform different functions than cells in the liver, but regardless of whether we are talking about cells that make up the heart, lungs, liver, or skin, all these cells share certain similarities. These similarities include cellular structures such as a membrane, mitochondria, and a nucleus. Importantly, for our discussion on cancer, each of our cells has another similarity: a cellular life cycle.

Cells go through three phases during their life cycle: interphase, mitosis, and cytokinesis. Interphase comprises the bulk of a cell's life. During interphase, each cell performs the functions in which it specializes, taking in nutrients, growing, synthesizing proteins, and ultimately preparing for mitosis. During mitosis, cells replicate their DNA, preparing to duplicate themselves. Finally, cells enter cytokinesis, at which point they split into two daughter cells, each containing identical copies of DNA.

DNA, or deoxyribonucleic acid, is the hereditary information contained inside every cell. DNA is contained within chromosomes.

Each cell has 46 chromosomes. We inherit 23 from mom, and 23 from dad. You can think of these chromosomes as your body's master code.

DNA is composed of chains made of four nucleotides: adenine, cytosine, thymine, and guanine. The way these four nucleotides are sequenced in chains is how information is coded into DNA, and this code is read by our body, similar to a computer reading binary code.

Segments of these nucleotide chains that comprise chromosomes are called genes. If you think of the four nucleotides as the ones and zeros in binary code, you can think of genes as specific, spelled-out commands for the body. We all know that genes control your physical appearance—traits such as height, eye color, and skin color, but genes control much more than this. Genes dictate functions right down to the cellular level, such as energy production in the cell and protein synthesis. These collections of genes make up individual chromosomes.

Our cells are particularly adept at replicating DNA during mitosis, as the continuation of life heavily relies on this being a reliable process! Overwhelmingly, DNA replication is extremely accurate. Remember, your body contains trillions of cells—all descendant from the united egg and sperm cells from mom and dad that merged to form a single cell—and even these trillions of cells are constantly replicating and replacing themselves.

Sometimes, though, mistakes can be made in the replication of DNA. Our cells do have methods for correcting these errors in replication when they happen, but sometimes they go undetected. Once any gene has been altered, it is known as a *mutation*. Subsequently, each daughter cell receives a copy of this mutated gene.

Genetic mutations are rare in the context of how many cells we have, and even when they do occur, they often occur in parts of the genetic code that do not control any sort of vital function and are subsequently unnoticed. However, genes control everything a cell does. Importantly, this includes a cell's lifecycle and division.

If enough mutations occur on specific genes, it is possible for cancer to form. Once cancer has formed, there traditionally have been six specific traits we have identified which distinguish cancerous cells from normal, healthy cells.

The first hallmark of cancerous cells is that they have self-sufficient growth signals. Whereas normal cells rely upon external signals to grow, cancer cells can stimulate themselves to grow and multiply.

Second, cancer cells do not respond to anti-growth signals the way normal cells do. Normal cells have what are known as *tumor-suppressor genes* which inhibit their growth. These tumor suppressor genes are altered in cancer cells, allowing the cancer cells to grow unchecked.

Third, cancer cells have the ability to evade programmed cell death, known as *apoptosis*. Apoptosis is a normal, healthy function in cells that have become "worn out." Cancer cells are immortal since they have lost their self-destruct mechanism.

Fourth, healthy cells have a predetermined number of times they can divide before dying, which is known as the *Hayflick limit*. Cancer cells have lost this pre-programmed function, allowing them to continue to multiply indefinitely.

The fifth hallmark of cancer is that cancer cells can promote *angiogenesis*, or the formation of new blood vessels to obtain nutrients, which cancer cells employ to nourish themselves to grow and ultimately spread. Normal cells cannot do this.

Finally, cancer cells invade nearby tissue and proliferate to different sites within the body, which is known as *metastasis*. (15)

These hallmarks were updated in 2011, to include two new additions. The first new hallmark of cancer proposed was deregulated metabolism. This simply means that cancer cells have a reprogrammed metabolism somewhat different from what we see in healthy cells, in order to promote cancer's continued growth and spread.

The second new hallmark is immune system evasion. This is based on the fact that cancer has ways of avoiding detection by the immune system, thus ensuring that it won't be attacked or eliminated by the body's natural defenses.

In addition to the two additional hallmarks, the 2011 paper also added two of what it calls "emerging characteristics." The first is what is known as *genomic instability*. This relates to random changes, or mutations, in cancer genes that tend to worsen as the cancer continues to grow and spread. These genetic changes can confer additional survival advantages to the cancer.

The second emerging characteristic added is inflammation. We know that inflammation is an irritation on the cellular level, and this plays a significant role in the formation and progression of cancer. (16)

Is Cancer a Genetic Disease or a Metabolic Disease?

With only a few exceptions, modern oncology maintains that cancer is purely a genetic disease. This is not unreasonable, because as we have just seen, genetic mutations precede the development of cancer. Thus, it is assumed that if you are dealt a bad genetic hand, invariably you are going to develop cancer at some point in your life, and there is not much you can do about it. This paradigm, which is known as the *somatic mutation theory*, has largely informed everything about the way cancer is treated today. However, this idea that cancer is purely genetic in origin might be somewhat short-sighted because it fails to address what lies at the root of genetic mutations to begin with.

The best data we have suggests that only between 6 and 8% of cancers are purely genetic in origin, meaning the incidence of cancer could solely be blamed on genes received from mom and dad. That leaves well over 90% of cancers with an unaccounted for etiology. Furthermore, in cases where there is a correlation between certain inherited genes, such as the BRCA1 and BRCA2 genes identified in cases of breast and ovarian cancer, the presence of those genes does not necessarily guarantee that cancer will form! Something simply does not add up when we look at cancer exclusively from a genetic standpoint.

I think that we are missing something upstream from the genetic abnormalities that we blame as being the cause of cancer. In other words, *something* caused these genetic abnormalities. Yes, we do see genetic abnormalities passed down from parents to children, but the genetic mutation you received from your grandma was likely the result of some sort of genetic insult that she incurred and passed on to her daughter, eventually resulting in cancer generations later.

As far as our understanding of what cancer is and how it forms, we have been the victims of our own success to some extent. As far as the standards of care are concerned, we have made massive leaps in the fields of radiology, chemotherapy, and surgery. Newer fields of immunotherapy are blossoming. These advancements have been made largely because we know more about genetics today than ever before. However, there is no doubt that our success in these fields has obscured inquiry into some of the more upstream causes of the genetic insults on which we blame cancer. We have focused so much on the genetic component of cancer that we have failed to see what sets those genetic changes in motion. This is important; if we can confidently assume that only 6–8% of cancers have a purely genetic origin, we must account for what is triggering the rise of cancers in over 90% of cancer cases.

The question becomes, what ultimately causes the genetic insults we see that give rise to cancer? I believe the answer to that question requires us to look at cancer from a different perspective. When we look at cancer as a metabolic disease instead of purely a genetic disease, many things about cancer begin to make more sense. Summarized simply, viewing cancer as a metabolic disease means that the genetic component of cancer is the result of our cell's metabolic processes—the process by which cells make energy—being interfered with and ultimately compromised by a variety of outside factors and/or agents.

We need another quick lesson in biology.

Adenosine triphosphate, or *ATP*, is the energy currency of our cells. ATP is produced by structures inside the cell known as *mitochondria*. ATP produced in the mitochondria supplies the entire cell with the energy necessary to carry out normal, healthy life processes.

Dr. Otto Warburg is a famous German scientist who was nominated for the Nobel Prize in medicine 46 times, a prize he won in 1931. Dr. Warburg did much to advance our understanding of cancer, and what ultimately won him the award was discovering how cancer cells made energy. According to Dr. Warburg, "The first phase (of cancer cells' origination) is the irreversible damage to respiration (metabolism)." (17)

Normal, healthy cells are good at producing ATP. Cells go through a multi-step process to produce energy that typically results in 32–36 units of ATP. Cancer cells, however, are not nearly as efficient; they typically only go through the first step of the metabolic process, known as *glycolysis*, wherein they metabolize glucose for energy. The result is only 2 units of ATP. This distinction between cancer cells and normal cells is very important.

Dr. Warburg would make other important discoveries related to cancer: He discovered that cancer cells can thrive in oxygen-poor environments and that cancer cells excrete lactic acid into their immediate environment. He was convinced, however, that this metabolic distinction between cancer cells and normal cells was paramount to understanding how cancer formed. He wrote:

> If the explanation of a vital process is its reduction to physics and chemistry, there is today no other explanation for the origin of cancer cells, either special or general. From this point of view, mutation and carcinogenic agents are not alternatives, but empty words, unless metabolically specified.

In other words, Dr. Warburg believed that genetic mutations were directly the result of compromised cellular metabolism. His research created a chicken-or-egg dilemma at the time, raising the question of which comes first: genetic changes or metabolic changes? If the somatic mutation theory is correct, the metabolic changes we see in cancer cells are a result of the DNA mutations that have occurred. However, if Warburg's metabolic theory of cancer is correct, the genetic changes we see in cancer cells occurs due to metabolic changes. This debate is still going on today.

With the discovery of chemotherapy in the 1940s, much of the thrust behind cancer research was put into developing therapeutic agents. While Dr. Warburg's research was cast aside for quite some time, there has been a revitalized interest in his discoveries which are now nearing 100 years old. Thankfully, many researchers are picking up where he left off. One of those researchers is Dr. Thomas Seyfried of Boston College.

Dr. Seyfried largely believes, as Dr. Warburg did, that cancer can be thought of as a metabolic disease as opposed to a genetic disease. In a study published in 2009, Dr. Seyfried says the following:

> All the major hallmarks of the disease (cancer) can be linked to impaired mitochondrial function . . . the abundance of somatic genomic abnormalities found in the majority of cancers can arise as a secondary consequence of mitochondrial dysfunction. Once established somatic genomic instability can contribute to further mitochondrial defects and to the metabolic inflexibility of the cancer cell. (18)

Dr. Seyfried believes that his research points toward the fact that the genetic abnormalities we associate with cancer are the direct result of interference with cellular metabolism. In his book *Cancer as a Metabolic Disease*, Dr. Seyfried summarizes an important study that sheds light on this idea.

Researchers took the nucleus of a cancer cell (remember that the nucleus is where all of the cell's genetic material is contained) and implanted it into an otherwise healthy cell. All of the other structures within the cell, such as the cellular membrane, the mitochondria, and the cytoplasm, were known to be healthy. To the surprise of most researchers, that cell with the cancerous nucleus did not go on to become cancerous itself. Simultaneously, researchers took the nucleus of a healthy cell and implanted it into a cell known to be cancerous. That cell went on and continued to be cancerous, even with the unhealthy genetic material replaced with healthy genetic material. (19)

The results of this study were shocking because it shook our fundamental understanding of what cancer is and how it forms. This knowledge, however, raises another important question: how does the metabolism of our cells become compromised to the point that genetic mutations occur and cancer forms?

The Toxic Bucket

Under normal circumstances, our cells endure a certain amount of insult and injury over the course of their lives. At a certain point, however, they can be overwhelmed and damaged by repeated bombardment. An analogy I like to use is that of a bucket. If you continue filling a bucket, eventually it will overflow.

Everyone in this analogy likely has a different-sized bucket. After all, some people can withstand cellular damage better than others. This explains why some people can smoke their entire lives and die of "natural" causes, while others might get lung cancer at a relatively young age. For all of us, though, a threshold likely exists. If our cells are bathed in a toxic environment for too long and/or they experience too many toxic hits, they become irreversibly damaged and can turn cancerous.

There are a variety of ways we can create toxic environments for our cells.

Carcinogens

Many people are familiar with the idea of carcinogens. *Carcinogens* are substances that are known or suspected of causing cancer. We are exposed to many of these carcinogens on a regular basis through our environment, the air we breathe, the food we eat, the things we drink, and even many of the consumer products we use, wear, or put on our skin.

Many of these are natural exposures. These include excessive amounts of UV radiation from the sun, or naturally occurring substances such as aflatoxins, radon, or asbestos silicate minerals. All of these are known to facilitate cancer formation. Even some infectious agents, such as the human papillomavirus (HPV) and the bacteria *H. pylori*, are known to cause cancer. This is important to remember, because often cancer is thought of as purely a disease of modernity, caused exclusively by man-made materials. In reality, we know that cancer has occurred in humans for as long as humans have existed, and natural exposures can be just as dangerous as man-made exposures.

Man-made exposures, of course, are a problem, too, and these include a wide variety of agents. Air pollution, certain pesticides, and certain agents used in industrial applications or consumer goods are all examples of man-made exposures that might play a role in the development of cancer. The number of these products thought to play a role in cancer seems to grow every day.

The International Agency for Research on Cancer (IARC) is an arm of the World Health Organization (WHO) tasked with identifying these carcinogenic agents. Their system includes a scaled, four-part classification system for categorizing substances that may contribute to cancer. Group 1 is known to be carcinogenic to humans. Group 2A is thought to be probably carcinogenic, while Group 2B is thought to possibly be carcinogenic. Group 3 represents substances that are undetermined as to whether or not they can cause cancer, and Group 4 are substances that are probably not carcinogenic.

The IARC has tested over 1,000 agents; of those agents, 120 belong to Group 1, 88 belong to Group 2A, 313 belong to Group 2B, and 499 belong to Group 3. This knowledge base is a good place to start, but it hardly scratches the surface of the myriad of chemical compounds that we come into contact with via our environment on a daily basis.

Ultimately, the likelihood of coming into contact with carcinogens in our environment is high, even for those who are the most mindful of their environment. The sum of all of these exposures can be thought of as filling our "toxic bucket," creating an environment for our cells that might not be ideal.

Lifestyle

When it comes to cancer, there is a marked lack of communication from the medical community to lay people in terms of the effect of lifestyle on the prevalence of cancer.

This is in stark contrast to diseases like heart disease and diabetes. The communication from the medical establishment to the general public concerning these two diseases has been consistent and clear for many years: If you want to avoid heart disease, do not smoke; enjoy alcohol in moderation; limit your intake of certain foods high in saturated fat; focus on fruits and vegetables; exercise regularly; avoid unhealthy fats. The advice for diabetes is largely the same.

Generally, however, this type of advice is not widely broadcast in terms of cancer. This is a problem, because there is no lack of evidence that lifestyle elements—such as diet, exercise, and mental/emotional health—play a significant role in cancer. Quite the contrary is true. In fact, some studies suggest that a majority of all cancers could be prevented with simple lifestyle changes. The implications of this are profound!

Sadly, the result of this lack of information regarding cancer is that most people aren't really aware of what actually causes cancer. Most people believe that getting cancer is just due to bad luck. When was the last time you heard someone say that about heart disease or diabetes?

If changes in lifestyle factors can prevent cancer, the corollary is also likely true: our lifestyle is likely facilitating the high incidence of cancers that we see in the developed world. We all know that we should exercise regularly, but many of us do not. We know that exercise benefits many aspects of health, including maintaining a healthy weight, improving cardiovascular fitness, and preventing cancer, yet the majority of people in the United States do not exercise. We all know that we should be eating more fruits and vegetables in lieu of processed foods, yet many people's diets are almost exclusively processed foods.

Increasingly, too, we are realizing that lifestyle factors like stress and proper sleep are crucial for maintaining our health. When these factors are neglected, the levels of cortisol—a hormone associated with stress—are raised. Cortisol is thought of as a bad thing, but its utility in the body is often misunderstood. Our bodies are adept at dealing with acute, immediate stressors—the types of events that initiated the fight-or-flight response that was necessary for our ancestors to survive the harsh conditions they endured before civilization made life more comfortable. When confronted by a predator or an enemy or when hunting food, our stress mechanisms allowed for sharp focus and feats of strength beyond what might be possible otherwise.

Our bodies are less adapted to the modern world, wherein we are subjected to constant, low-level stress: traffic on a freeway, a deadline at work, or unresolved emotional trauma. The result is a constant, low-level flood of stress hormones that ultimately have negative effects on our health. In a way, these stress mechanisms which were designed to keep us safe and help us survive have been co-opted by the modern lifestyle that was supposed to make our lives easier. Now, they might be working more toward our detriment than our good.

Malignancy in Order to Survive

The result of all of these factors, including toxic environmental exposures and poor lifestyle factors, is inflammation. Particularly in the last few decades, researchers have discovered that inflammation plays a key role in many of the chronic diseases that people experience, including cancer.

We know that when our cells are inflamed, they are less efficient and do not work as well as they otherwise should. This cumulative inflammation ultimately creates a situation wherein our cells are so damaged that they must mutate in order to survive. This is the toxic bucket "overflowing."

This is a very simplified way to understand cancer as a metabolic disease. After all, an entire book could be written on the scientific details. For our purposes here, know that inflammation creates a cellular environment wherein our cells do not function as they should, which impedes their ability to create energy, and ultimately leads to the genetic insults that set cancer formation in motion.

Genetics vs. Epigenetics

In large part, it is likely that such a void exists in the greater discussion about cancer prevention because for too long, we have thought about cancer mostly as a disease of genetic bad luck. If you are unfortunate enough to have been dealt a bad genetic hand, then you have little say over whether or not you will get cancer during your lifetime, or at least that is what we have been led to believe.

The paradigm I have laid out, however—one in which cancer can be thought of as a metabolic disease as opposed to simply a genetic disease—gives us some hope in this regard. Viewing cancer in this way means that we do have significant control over our risk of cancer and factors within our control can be used in a positive way to fight cancer. When we combine this with the fact that less than 10% of cancers are purely genetic in origin, the idea that we are solely at the will of the genetic hand we are dealt begins to fall apart.

Certainly, our genes control a number of factors about ourselves that are out of control. You can't change your height, the color of your eyes, the color of your hair, or other factors that are directly controlled by your genetics. The genes you inherit from mom and dad control much about you, but the idea that your genes control your cancer risk with absolute authority is not totally founded on what the most recent research tells us. In fact, a rapidly emerging field of study is calling into question much of what we thought we knew about genetics.

Epigenetics is an exciting area of research that seeks to understand how our genes—the information written into the genetic material of all of our cells—interact with their environment and ultimately change or react as a result of the environment in which they are immersed. It is only recently that we have discovered that our genes—far from being written in stone—are reacting to their environment as often as on an hourly basis.

This has enormous implications for the idea that "bad" genes bear the exclusive responsibility for poor genetic outcomes. With the exception of some very specific and rare genetic diseases, we have learned that bad genes, such as the genes responsible for causing cancer or other disease thought to be associated closely with genetics, can be turned on or off depending on the environment they are in.

How do we influence the cellular environment that affects our genes? Simply put, the myriad of factors that we collectively dub as our *lifestyle* hold enormous influence over this cellular environment. Everything from the air we breathe, toxic environmental exposures, and even factors like stress and emotional health can have an influence on the cellular level, ultimately influencing our genes in a negative or positive way.

One of the most important epigenetic factors that has been studied, however, is diet. It is known that many nutrients inherent in certain foods can help prevent cancer, and it turns out that the reason these foods might provide cancer-protective properties might have much to do with the epigenetic effects these nutrients facilitate. (20, 21)

The science of epigenetics is new and emerging, but the direction in which it is pointing has enormous implications for cancer as well as many other diseases. In a sense, our genetics might "load the gun," rendering some of us susceptible to certain types of cancer. Lifestyle, however, is what "pulls the trigger." This makes lifestyle a powerful preventative tool.

While much research has been conducted on the effects certain foods might have on cancer incidence or prevention, much of the emerging research reveals that it is not just what we eat, but how we structure our eating, which can have desirable anti-cancer effects. Specifically, enduring periods of fasting might be a powerful, heretofore untapped strategy for cancer prevention and as a modality for treatment. In this book, we hope to underscore some of that research while also explaining what fasting is and how to incorporate it into your life so you may experience abundant health.

References

(1) "Lifetime Risk of Developing or Dying From Cancer." *American Cancer Society*, www.cancer.org/cancer/cancer-basics/lifetime-probability-of-developing-or-dying-from-cancer.html.

(2) "Early History of Cancer." American Cancer Society. N.p., n.d. Web. 26 July 2017.

(3) "History of Breast Cancer." *Senology*. N.p., n.d. Web. 26 July 2017.

(4) "Science Diction: The Origin of the Word 'Cancer'." *NPR*. NPR, 22 Oct. 2010. Web. 26 July 2017.

(5) Olszewski, Margaret M., PhD. "Concepts of Cancer from Antiquity to the Nineteenth Century." *University of Toronto Medical Journal.* 87.3 (May 2010): n. pag. Web. 25 July 2017.

(6) Bray F, Ferlay J, Soerjomataram I, et al. "Global Cancer Statistics 2018: GLOBOCAN Estimates of Incidence and Mortality Worldwide for 36 Cancers in 185 Countries." *CA Cancer J Clin* 2018; 68(6): 394-424. doi: 10.3322/caac.21492.

(7) "Cancer." *World Health Organization*, World Health Organization, www.who.int/en/news-room/fact-sheets/detail/cancer.

(8) "Cancer Statistics." *National Cancer Institute*, www.cancer.gov/about-cancer/understanding/statistics.

(9) Siegel R.L., Miller K.D., Wagle N.S., and Jemal A. "Cancer Statistics, 2023." *CA Cancer J Clin* 2023; 73(1): 17-48. doi: 10.3322/caac.21763.

(10) Jones, David S., MD, PhD, Scott H. Podolsky, MD, and Jeremy A. Greene, MD, PhD. "The Burden of Disease and the Changing Task of Medicine." *New England Journal of Medicine.* 366.25 (2012): 2333-338. Web. 29 June 2017.

(11) Ahmad, A.S., N.O. Smith, and P.D. Sasieni. "Trends in the Lifetime Risk of Developing Cancer in Great Britain: Comparison of Risk for Those Born from 1930 to 1960." *British Journal of Cancer* 112 (2015): n. pag. Web. 29 June 2017.

(12) "Study Finds Sharp Rise in Colon Cancer and Rectal Cancer Rates Among Young Adults." *American Cancer Society. N.p., n.d. Web. 02 July 2017.*

(13) Balar, Dr. Bhavesh. "The Three Reasons so Many People Are Getting Cancer (Op-Ed)." *LiveScience*, Purch, 5 June 2015,

www.livescience.com/51099-the-three-reasons-cancer-rates-are-rising.html.

(14) "Facts & Figures 2019: US Cancer Death Rate Has Dropped 27% in 25 Years." *American Cancer Society*, www.cancer.org/latest-news/facts-and-figures-2019.html.

(15) Hanahan D, Weinberg R.A. "The Hallmarks of Cancer." *Cell* 2000 Jan 7; 100 (1): 57-70.

(16) Hanahan D., Weinberg R.A. Hallmarks of Cancer: The Next Generation. *Cell* 2011; 144(5): 646-74. doi:10.1016/j.cell.2011.02.013.

(17) Warburg, Otto H. "On the Origin of Cancer Cells." *Science* 123.3191 (1956): 309-14. Print.

(18) Seyfried, Thomas N., and Laura M. Shelton. "Cancer as a Metabolic Disease." *Nutrition & Metabolism* 7.1 (2010): 7. Web.

(19) Seyfried, Thomas N. "Cancer as a Mitochondrial Metabolic Disease." *Frontiers in Cell and Developmental Biology*, vol. 3, July 2015, doi:10.3389/fcell.2015.00043.

(20) Arora I., Sharma M., and Tollefsbol TO. "Combinatorial Epigenetics Impact of Polyphenols and Phytochemicals in Cancer Prevention and Therapy." *Int J Mol Sci* 2019; 20(18): 4567. doi: 10.3390/ijms20184567.

(21) Shankar E., Kanwal R., Candamo M., and Gupta S. "Dietary Phytochemicals as Epigenetic Modifiers in Cancer: Promise and Challenges." *Semin Cancer Biol* 2016; 40-41: 82-99. doi: 10.1016/j.semcancer.2016.04.002.

CHAPTER 2

An Introduction to Fasting

I saw few die of hunger; of eating, a hundred thousand.
— BENJAMIN FRANKLIN

Three square meals a day.

For the majority of us, eating three meals a day has been the expectation our entire lives. You eat breakfast when you wake up. Halfway through the day you enjoy lunch. After a long day at work, school, or taking care of your family, you eat dinner before bed. This rhythm has largely dictated how the schedule for our entire society is laid out. Work days are oriented around the times we are supposed to eat, as are school days. Restaurants open for breakfast, lunch, or dinner, or a combination of all three. The pace of our modern world, hectic though it may be, is punctuated by mealtimes. The ability to enjoy three square meals a day is seen as a metric for discerning poverty or wealth in a society. These three meals—breakfast, lunch, and dinner—spaced out over the day, is a deeply ingrained societal construct.

It wasn't always this way, however.

No doubt, the idea of orienting our entire schedule around mealtimes, which are spaced out over the course of the day, is a vestige we have inherited from past societies. But on the scale of time that humans have roamed the earth, this idea of orienting our days around specific mealtimes over the course of the day is a newer concept. Our ancestors, particularly before the advent of agriculture, did not always have the luxury of deciding when they ate—or even how often they ate. By no choice of their own, they were forced into periods of not being able to eat anything at all, otherwise known as *fasting*. Yet despite these difficult circumstances, they survived, and the human race flourished.

Today, however, we enjoy an abundance of food that is greater than anything man has ever known. Particularly in wealthy societies, the idea of food scarcity is largely a thing of the past. Many of us have only ever experienced an abundance of food, rather than a complete lack of it.

Furthermore, those three meals that are the baseline expectation in a developed society are often punctuated by snacking whenever you feel like it. In today's world, all barriers preventing us from consuming calories have been removed. We can eat virtually whatever we want, whenever we want it. And many, if not most of us, do.

In some respects, abundance is a good thing. Having more than enough food on hand to eliminate the worry of starvation is an incredible privilege. In many ways, this urge to have a steady, constant, and reliable source of food is what has driven the development of civilization over millennia. And still today, there are parts of the world where this sort of bounty would be an enormous answer to prayer. We truly are very blessed.

However, we must acknowledge that there are some unintended consequences associated with the bounty we are so fortunate to enjoy.

As we discussed in chapter 1, we know that we are facing a health crisis as a society. In addition to cancer, we know heart disease, diabetes, and obesity are rampant. Some grim statistics about health in America provide us a harrowing perspective:

- 69% of adults are overweight, with 36.5% of adults being considered obese. In addition, 17% of children ages 2–19 are considered obese, while 12.5% of preschoolers are obese. (1)
- 26.8 million people in the United States have been diagnosed as diabetic, representing 10.2% of the population. It is estimated that at least an additional 7.3 million people have diabetes but have not yet received a formal diagnosis. (2)
- In 2017, 868,662 people died from heart disease. Between 2015 and 2018, 126.9 million Americans had some form of cardiovascular disease. (3)
- According to data collected from 2015 to 2017, 39.5% of men and women can expect to be diagnosed with cancer at some point in their lives. (4)

Unfortunately, there is little encouraging data that suggests these diseases will do anything but become more prevalent in the coming years. The logical question is, what do these diseases have to do with our diet?

The role of diet in disease is a notoriously tricky thing to study. We are heavily reliant upon what people report, which is not always the most reliable data. It is even more difficult to study one particular food and discern whether that food is good, bad, or neither, or possibly both. There is simply a myriad of factors that come into play when evaluating how nutrition affects our health.

What we can do, however, is study dietary trends—take a bird's-eye view, so to speak—and correlate those trends with disease incidence. In addition, we can look at smaller studies in humans and animals to discern how dietary changes affect biochemistry and physiology. We still have much to learn, but we know more today than ever before. Thus, we can also confidently say with a high degree of certainty that *what* we eat plays a significant role in the prevalence of diseases like cancer, heart disease, and diabetes. This is well-documented in the literature:

- There is abundant evidence that dietary modifications can prevent diabetes, and even those who have already been diagnosed with diabetes can often manage their disease with changes in diet. A Mediterranean diet that focuses on whole, plant foods is recommended. (5)
- Similarly, it is thought that heart disease, which is the number one cause of death worldwide in developed countries, could largely be prevented by focusing on fruits, vegetables, legumes, whole grains, and nuts. (6)
- Studies have shown that cancer rates could be cut in half with simple lifestyle changes, including a better diet. (7) That is a profound statistic in a society where roughly 40% of people are currently expected to develop cancer. Furthermore, people who eat healthier diets fare better in terms of treatment outcomes as well as in mitigation of treatment-related side effects. (8)

We can confidently say that the right type of diet can help prevent chronic diseases. The opposite is also true: poor diet can be a contributing factor in the prevalence of these diseases.

Most of the research done on the relationship between diet and disease has focused on the types and quality of food that people eat—*what* we eat. Subsequently, much of the conversation about diet has centered around what we eat. Most of us are keenly aware by now that fresh fruits, vegetables, legumes, whole grains, nuts, and seeds are the foods on which we should focus. As we will discuss later in the book, what we eat is very important in our fight against cancer and other diseases. Time and time again, these are the foods that show up in the research as being the foods that help support health and vitality. Furthermore, it is true that eliminating highly processed foods, including ingredients such as added sugars, colors, flavors, dyes, preservatives, and unhealthy fats, is a step in the right direction.

However, we are painting an incomplete picture if we focus only on *what* we eat, while ignoring *how much* and *how often* we eat.

One example of how simply focusing on the quality of the foods you eat can be shortsighted is the myriad experiments conducted wherein participants lose weight while only eating unhealthy foods such as desserts and processed foods. When participants in such experiments keep their total calorie intake below the calories they burn throughout the day, they still lose weight. In some cases, lab testing showed improvements in several markers we commonly associate with good health. This goes against what most of us think when it comes to nutrition, and it certainly would horrify most nutritionists, doctors, nurses, and other health professionals. It does, however, reveal an important yet simple truth: When it comes to nutrition's impact on your health, how much you eat might matter as much as what you eat.

Being overweight or obese dramatically increases the risk of many kinds of diseases, including cancer. (9) But if you can control your weight while technically eating all the "wrong" foods, thus diminishing some of the health risks posed by being overweight, this might be a clue that we have only been focusing on part of the picture.

We can say with certainty, without even beginning to address the quality of the foods that we eat, that most of us simply eat *too much*.

There are many reasons why we eat too much. Some people eat for comfort or for entertainment. Some people eat too fast, ignoring or missing the body's hormonal signals that tell us when we've had enough to eat. Some people—by the nature of the calorically dense, nutritionally void, processed foods they live on—simply eat too many calories. It is likely that the majority of people eat in a way that is the opposite of mindful. In other words, we eat whatever we want, whenever we want it, eating out of pure desire, habit, or boredom, with little regard for whether it is truly beneficial for our health or necessary for our daily nourishment.

There is no doubt that how much and how often we eat is largely informed by the abundance and availability of food we enjoy. We as a society have removed all barriers to obtaining food. For most people, overeating is an unintended consequence of the abundance we enjoy. When we couple this with the addictive nature of many of the processed foods available, it is not difficult to see how this can have catastrophic effects on our health.

This is where the idea of fasting might have some profound benefits.

Let's revisit that image of our ancestors in a pre-agricultural revolution world, who are largely considered to have been hunter-gatherers. By nature of their circumstances, they would have necessarily endured periods wherein there was no food. Between hunts, or in the winter months when wild plants which provided food were scarce, there would be periods of consuming no calories. Their bodies would have been forced into a state of fasting.

If this fasted state rendered our ancestors incapable of performing basic tasks, with little to no energy or ability to focus, that would have been extremely disadvantageous. With other predators to contend with, this would have been a very dangerous situation that compromised survival.

Interestingly, emerging research indicates that our bodies are actually designed to deal with a fasted state quite well. Instead of brain fog, fasted states can facilitate mental sharpness. Instead of lethargy, energy can increase. Down to the cellular level, there are benefits to fasting that the majority of the modern world routinely misses due to how we typically eat.

So what does this mean for us today? In a time when we have an abundance of food at our fingertips whenever we desire it, how do we incorporate this idea of *not eating* in a meaningful, healthy way? Does fasting have any place in the twenty-first century?

On the surface, fasting seems to go against everything our brains are hardwired to do. Food is not only pleasurable; it is necessary and vital to our survival, our health, and our well-being. Yet research tells us that fasting can have profound benefits for our health. In particular, fasting might have some profound benefits for our fight against cancer. Whether you are looking to prevent cancer or you have been diagnosed with cancer, you can glean some tremendous benefits from regularly forcing your body into a fasted state.

What Is Fasting?

The simplest and perhaps most accurate description of fasting is that it is the restriction or elimination of calories for certain periods of time. Even more simply put, fasting is not eating. While this is a profoundly simple concept, there is some confusion, mostly in terms of how the word *fasting* is used. It is not uncommon to hear people say they are fasting from sugar or processed foods. You might have even heard people say they are fasting from technology, or things like television or social media. In the sense that you are restricting or altogether eliminating these things, there is some similarity to fasting. True fasting, however, is not consuming any sort of calories.

It helps to clear up some confusion about some of the other ways the word *fasting* is misused as it relates to diet. Often, in an attempt to modulate their health or lose weight, people will say they are going on a "juice fast," wherein they eliminate all food except freshly-squeezed fruit and vegetable juices for a period of time. Similarly, a "broth fast" consists of relying solely on bone broth or vegetable broth for a specified amount of time. In these cases, the "fast" usually lasts anywhere from a single day to several days. The problem with thinking of this as fasting is that you are still consuming calories. Remember, true fasting does not involve consuming any calories whatsoever.

Another point we must clarify is that fasting is not the same as starvation. Indeed, fasting means that you are eliminating calories for a certain period of time, and when that time is over, you eat. Certainly, if you went too long without eating, you would become malnourished.

If you remained malnourished for long enough, you would approach the point of starvation. The kind of fasting we are discussing will not approach starvation or even malnutrition—ever.

Similar to the fact that fasting is not starvation, it is important to realize that fasting is not necessarily about deprivation either. Fasting is about organizing the times when you permit yourself to eat and the times you do not eat. Fasting itself does not necessarily inform what you should eat during the times you are permitting yourself to eat. What you eat, of course, is important as well, which is something we will discuss later in the book. Fasting, however, is not a diet, and it is not about starving yourself. Rather, fasting is simply about eliminating any sort of caloric consumption for certain, extended periods of time.

Finally, fasting is not an eating disorder. Eating disorders, such as anorexia or bulimia, are serious conditions with deep psychological roots and obvious clinical consequences. Fasting is neither forced starvation nor intentional deprivation. Fasting is a way of organizing when you eat. An important delineation between fasting and eating disorders is the consequences for our health. Eating disorders invariably detract from health, whereas fasting—when done appropriately—works to elevate our health. While fasting can help people lose unwanted weight, its benefits and utility extend far beyond just fat loss or chasing a desired body image. Furthermore, for those who do not want to lose weight (especially in the case of cancer patients suffering from cachexia), it is entirely possible to glean the benefits of fasting without using it as a modality to lose weight.

We now have a clearer idea about what fasting is: the intentional restriction of calories for periods of time, with the purpose of optimizing our health.

A Brief History of Fasting

Fasting as a practice has existed for as long as humans have. As we discussed previously, our ancestors were forced into periods of fasting as they roamed the earth in search of food. While food scarcity would have been a constant issue, clearly it did not deter the human race from flourishing. Research suggests that the fasted state not only happened with regularity, but that it was integral to our development as a species.

With the emergence of the agricultural revolution, humans were able to develop permanent settlements and more complex societies. Interestingly, the practice of fasting—once a state that was forced by circumstances—continued as these societies advanced.

Fasting has largely been part of religious and cultural practices throughout human history. Interestingly, fasting developed independently throughout cultures worldwide. (10) This is noteworthy, because people in antiquity were heavily reliant on their senses and observation. It is interesting to think that many ancient remedies such as herbal medicines are now today being confirmed by scientific studies as having benefits. I believe that fasting is similar in that regard. Our ancestors in antiquity likely noticed there was some benefit to fasting and thus incorporated the practice into their societies.

The ancient Greeks, including Pythagoras, Abaris, and Epimenides, extolled the benefits of fasting. During that time, fasting was often used as a means of preparing for religious rituals. (10) In the Hellenistic religions, the gods were only thought to reveal their divine revelations to people who had participated in fasting. In pre-Columbian Peru, fasting was used as a penance for sins confessed to a priest. Native Americans incorporated fasting into their rituals, often fasting before or during vision quests. Religions throughout the world have used fasting as a means to assuage angry deities or as a means of supplication for bountiful harvests, victories in war, or other requests to the divine. (11)

Perhaps most familiar for many people is the myriad of ways that fasting was used in the Bible. Fasting is referenced throughout both the Old and New Testaments, from Moses, to Jesus, and to the disciples. It was used as a tool for a variety of purposes, including the following:

- Preparation for ministry
- A modality for seeking God's wisdom
- An act of grief
- Supplication for deliverance, protection, or victory in some form of battle
- A form of repentance
- An act of worship (12)

Perhaps the most famous reference to fasting is when Jesus fasted in the desert for 40 days and 40 nights in preparation for his ministry, just prior to being tempted by Satan.

With such an emphasis on fasting throughout the Bible, I am hard-pressed as a Christian not to see significance in the practice and the application of fasting in our lives today. If fasting is a practice that is so purposefully included in the Bible, surely it is something God would have us incorporate into our lives for spiritual reasons. Yet, like many practices which facilitate spiritual health, science has also identified benefits to our physical, mental, and emotional health.

Take prayer, for example. Some studies indicate that taking time for prayer each day can have significant benefits for stress reduction, which ultimately supports our physical and emotional health. Fasting, it seems—even if you are only participating in fasting for spiritual purposes—likely confers physical benefits as well. Almost invariably, this was something our ancestors noticed.

A Brief History of Fasting for Therapeutic Benefits

As far back as the 5th century BC, the Greeks recognized the therapeutic benefits of fasting. Hippocrates, considered the father of medicine, was a proponent of fasting. He wrote, "To eat when you are sick is to feed your illness." Other Greek thinkers who were proponents of fasting as a form of medicinal treatment were Plutarch, Plato, and Aristotle. The Greeks observed that when animals were sick, they would naturally forgo food. They reasoned if animals fasted when they felt ill, perhaps it was a good practice for humans to do the same. (13)

More about the physiological effects of fasting began to be understood in the 19th century. Around this time, our understanding of human nutritional requirements was greatly expanded, and more modern forms of scientific study were used to examine how the body responded to fasting. As more was understood, modified methods of fasting began to be employed. (11) Some of these are still useful today, which we will discuss in later chapters. During this time, fasting was studied for a variety of issues; among them (perhaps most obviously) was weight loss. In one extreme example, under the watchful eye of physicians, a severely obese 27-year-old man fasted for 382 days and lost an enormous 272 pounds.

While today there is a revitalized interest in the idea of fasting, the idea of using fasting to achieve specific ends is nothing new. From antiquity, our ancestors have realized that fasting brings with it many benefits, and while they may not have known exactly how or why fasting was beneficial, today we have the scientific insight to better understand how fasting works, what the best ways are to incorporate fasting into our lives, and what we can reasonably expect from fasting.

It is important to remember that there is no such thing as a silver bullet in medicine, or for our health. With that said, we will see in future chapters that fasting shows much promise for a wide variety of health conditions, including cancer. If you are interested in elevating your health, you should at the very least consider incorporating fasting into your regimen.

Who Should and Who Should Not Fast

Fasting is an enormous departure from the way many of us are accustomed to eating. In addition to the expectation of three meals a day, many people snack whenever they feel like it. To begin integrating fasting into our lifestyles simply constitutes an enormous change for most people, and most people will find it to be a difficult habit to form.

There is, however, a growing body of evidence which suggests that integrating fasting into our modern lifestyle provides some profound benefits. Our focus for the rest of this book will be to examine the benefits associated with fasting as they relate to cancer. The benefits of fasting, however, are not limited to its direct anticancer effects. Fasting has also been shown to improve metabolism, lower blood sugar, reduce inflammation, help detoxify the body, and assist in removing damaged cells. (14) If you are familiar with my integrative oncology practice, you can already begin to see how these proven benefits have profound implications for our fight against cancer. We will discuss these benefits, as well as how to incorporate fasting into your lifestyle, which types of fasts might be the most beneficial, what happens when you fast, and what to eat when you are not fasting so as to maximally support your health by creating an anticancer environment within your body.

Like all good things, however, fasting can be done incorrectly, and if you are not careful, fasting improperly can bring with it the risk of certain health problems. One of the most acute risks associated with fasting is dehydration. It is imperative to drink sufficient amounts of water, whether you are fasting or not. Remember that water has zero calories, and drinking water does not constitute breaking your fast. There are people who have abstained from drinking water as part of a fast, but this is not recommended, nor is there any scientific information to support the idea of fasting from water. You need hydration, *especially* if you are fasting. I recommend that people drink at least half of their body weight in ounces of water daily. For example, if you weigh 150 pounds, strive to drink at least 75 ounces of water (approximately 2.2 liters) per day.

Longer fasts can be beneficial in the right setting for the right patient, but the longer the fast, the more elevated the risk for complications or adverse side effects. Although we referenced the incredible account of a man losing 272 pounds by fasting for over a year, this was done in a clinical setting under the guidance of physicians highly trained in therapeutic fasting. And while the man didn't eat any food, his intake of certain nutrients was supplemented. Failure to do so would have been dangerous and ultimately life-threatening.

This is a good time to point out that even natural remedies can have serious unintended consequences. This underscores the importance of working with your doctor when trying a new diet, supplement, or even fasting regimen. As an integrative oncologist, one of my jobs is to sift through the research pertaining to natural, holistic, and "alternative" remedies, in addition to learning about the cutting-edge research within the conventional oncology community. Unfortunately, we live in an age where pseudoscience, misinformation, and information that is flat-out wrong gets perpetuated and promoted, particularly online. It has never been easier to educate yourself on any subject, but that doesn't mean you are getting *good* information. With my medical training, years of clinical experience, and expertise, I'm in a good place to evaluate the available evidence and ultimately discern which treatments and protocols are backed by solid science and might carry some benefit for my patients—hence the penning of this book. The evidence emerging regarding the benefits of fasting, particularly for our fight against cancer, leads to me to believe this information constitutes an invaluable tool. I believe this information is important enough to relay to the general public.

It is important to remember that no amount of self-education takes the place of the formal education and clinical experience of a physician. However, most physicians are not trained in therapeutic fasting, so they are not aware of many of the details in this book. With that said, please discuss any dietary or supplement changes you make with your physician, particularly if you are taking any medications or undergoing any form of treatment for any type of disease. If your physician cannot adequately help you, please find one who can.

As far as fasting is concerned, certain individuals may not be good candidates for fasting. This includes the following:

- Women who are pregnant or nursing.
- Those who have impaired blood glucose regulation, especially diabetics who use insulin.
- Individuals with high blood pressure, heart disease, or who are prone to electrolyte abnormalities.
- Those who have suffered from eating disorders such as bulimia or anorexia. (14, 15)

Please consult with your physician before moving forward with any sort of fasting protocol, *especially* if you fall into one of the categories listed above. In addition, it is generally not recommended for children or adolescents to fast except under extreme circumstances and under the watchful eye of an expert.

However, if you are otherwise healthy, it is very likely that you can safely incorporate fasting into your regimen. I believe that fasting is something we should all be trying to incorporate into our routines. In tandem with a nutrition plan, exercise, stress reduction, and getting enough sleep on a regular basis, fasting helps round out healthy lifestyle factors and puts us in the best position to not just prevent and/or fight cancer, but to enjoy a life of abundant health.

References

(1) Holland, K. (2020, July 29). Retrieved June 7, 2021, from https://www.healthline.com/health/obesity-facts#2.-Obesity-affects-1-in-6-children-in-the-United-States.

(2) (n.d.). Retrieved June 7, 2021, from https://www.diabetesresearch.org/diabetes-statistics.

(3) Virani S.S., Alonso A., Aparicio H.J., et al. on behalf of the American Heart Association Council on Epidemiology and Prevention Statistics Committee and Stroke Statistics Subcommittee. *Heart Disease and Stroke Statistics—2021 Update: A Report from the American Heart Association* [published online ahead of print January 27, 2021]. *Circulation.* doi: 10.1161/CIR.0000000000000950.

(4) "Cancer Statistics." (n.d.). Retrieved from https://www.cancer.gov/about-cancer/understanding/statistics.

(5) Asif, M. (2014). "The Prevention and Control of Type-2 Diabetes by Changing Lifestyle and Dietary Pattern." *Journal of Education and Health Promotion, 3*(1), 1. doi:10.4103/2277-9531.127541.

(6) Yu, E., Malik, V. S., & Hu, F. B. (2018). "Cardiovascular Disease Prevention by Diet Modification: JACC Health Promotion Series." *Journal of the American College of Cardiology, 72*(8), 914-926. doi:10.1016/j.jacc.2018.02.085.

(7) Song, Mingyang, and Edward Giovannucci. "Preventable Incidence and Mortality of Carcinoma Associated with Lifestyle Factors Among White Adults in the United States." *JAMA Oncology* 2.9 (2016): 1154. Web.

(8) Collective, The Tincture. "Nutrition and Cancer: Where Do We Go from Here? – Tincture." *Tincture* 4 Mar. 2016, tincture.io/nutrition-and-cancer-where-do-we-go-from-here-7f93632e0464. Accessed 21 Aug. 2017.

(9) Obesity and Cancer Fact Sheet. (n.d.). Retrieved from https://www.cancer.gov/about-cancer/causes-prevention/risk/obesity/obesity-fact-sheet.

(10) Kerndt, P.R., Naughton, J.L., Driscoll, C.E., & Loxterkamp, D.A. (1982). "Fasting: The History, Pathophysiology and Complications." *Western Journal of Medicine,* 137(5), 379-399. Retrieved June 7, 2021.

(11) "Fasting." (n.d.). Retrieved from https://www.britannica.com/topic/fasting.

(12) Feola, K. (2021, February 17). "Why Should I Fast? 7 Examples of Fasting in the Bible." Retrieved from https://www.faithgateway.com/why-should-i-fast-7-examples-fasting-bible/#.YKQXPi2cZ24.

(13) "Fasting – A History Part I." (2021, April 07). Retrieved from https://thefastingmethod.com/fasting-a-history-part-i/.

(14) Monique Tello, M. (2018, June 29). "Intermittent Fasting: Surprising Update." Retrieved from https://www.health.harvard.edu/blog/intermittent-fasting-surprising-update-2018062914156.

(15) "Not So Fast: Pros and Cons of the Newest Diet Trend." (2019, July 31). Retrieved from https://www.health.harvard.edu/heart-health/not-so-fast-pros-and-cons-of-the-newest-diet-trend.

CHAPTER 3

From Feasting to Fasting

What Happens to Your Body When You Fast

Because fasting has been studied in a scientific and medical capacity for more than a century, we have a good idea about what happens inside our bodies when we fast. And because fasting is all about timing when you eat, it helps to have a good understanding of the changes that will occur in the body on a timeline following your last meal.

Preparation for Fasting

Certainly, many people have some anxiety about beginning a fasting regimen. After all, it has been ingrained into us that we should eat three times a day, every day, and snack in between. The biggest question when it comes to fasting is, of course, "What if I get hungry?"

The short answer is, you will, especially in the beginning.

Hunger, however, is not always a sign that you must eat immediately or experience dire health consequences. Many people falsely assume that the feeling of hunger is immediately derived from an empty stomach. In other words, most of us think when we eat, our stomach fills up and tells our brains we are full; when it empties, we become hungry. This is not entirely accurate; in fact, hunger is a hormonal signal which can be cued by things other than just the need to eat.

Have you ever walked by a bakery or into your favorite restaurant and immediately felt your stomach growl? Have you ever seen a picture of a perfectly plated meal or a wedding cake being cut and immediately felt a craving for something delicious? Sometimes, it is obvious when our hunger is stimulated by things other than the need to eat.

Also, if you are like many people and you have a daily routine of eating three meals at approximately the same times most days out of the week, your body is very much adapted to eating at those specific times, and right around breakfast time, you will start feeling that gnawing of hunger in your stomach. This is to be expected, but does it really mean you *must* eat at this moment?

As we will learn, from a metabolic perspective, there is no reason to assume that we need three meals a day, placed at certain times throughout the day. Nor must you frequently snack to "maintain your blood sugar." These are largely myths that most people mistake for nutritional truth. The reality is our body is well-designed to deal with a fasted state.

As you begin your fasting regimen, it is important to realize that the hunger you experience does not mean that you must eat. If you have been cleared by your doctor to begin a fasting regimen or if you are otherwise healthy, you will learn that your body actually benefits from periods of not eating, but particularly in the beginning, we must learn to control our hunger. At first, it can be uncomfortable, but know that after a certain period of time, most people report their hunger diminishes, that they wind up eating less while feeling totally satisfied. When feelings of hunger do arise, they are no longer overwhelming and may be a truer indication that your body requires fuel.

Your Final Meal to a Fasted State

The time has come for your final meal. For our purposes, we are going to assume that you are eating a balanced meal containing approximately equal parts of fats, carbohydrates, and protein. This is noteworthy, simply because our bodies process these different macronutrients—which are the body's three primary sources of fuel—in different ways.

Most of us need approximately 2,000 calories a day to maintain our body's basal metabolic rate and supply the energy needed for going about our daily lives. *Basal metabolic rate*, or *BMR*, is the sum of all the calories needed to both get up and move around like we normally would and fuel the chemical reactions and processes that keep us alive; all of these things require energy to take place. Some of these are processes we normally would not even think about, things like our heart continuing to beat, breathing, or the myriad of processes going on inside the body that none of us consciously make happen, yet they are critical for sustaining our life.

A normal meal might consist of anywhere between 400 and 800 calories. So invariably you consume more calories than you immediately need whenever you eat; those calories are not immediately used. So what happens to them? Because all of the calories we consume in a sitting are not immediately used as fuel, our body must store this extra energy somehow. During digestion, carbohydrates are broken down quickly into glucose, the form of sugar found in the blood. Proteins are broken down into amino acids, and many of these amino acids are absorbed for use in building and repairing structures in the body. Excess amino acids, however, are converted into glucose as well. As glucose in the body increases, it prompts the rise of an important hormone: insulin.

Insulin is the hormone necessary for two very important tasks: helping our body use the energy from food and storing excess energy from food.

In the first capacity, as glucose levels become elevated in the blood after we eat, insulin helps usher glucose into each of the cells in our body so they can burn it as energy. Most people have a negative connotation surrounding glucose, or "blood sugar"; we think of it as a bad thing, but in reality, glucose is one of our cells' primary sources of fuel. Without fuel, our cells will die. Glucose is very important in this regard!

Insulin also assists in storing excess glucose not immediately used by our cells; this is so the body has energy on hand. Excess glucose is first converted to glycogen, which is stored in the liver. Glycogen is used as energy when blood sugar levels begin to drop. The liver keeps a certain amount of glycogen on hand, but there is a limit to how much of it the liver can store. Once the liver is at capacity for glycogen, any excess glucose is converted to fat and then deposited throughout the body. While the liver has limits on glycogen, there is virtually no limit on the amount of fat that can be stored throughout the body.

Dietary fats are absorbed directly by the body and do not have an effect on insulin levels.

To recap: When you eat, your blood sugar rises, which prompts a rise in insulin. Any excess glucose is first stored as glycogen in the liver, and once the liver is at capacity, glucose is stored as fat.

Now, the fasting begins.

Remember, fasting is simply not consuming any calories, which results in the above processes we just discussed.

Naturally, as you begin fasting, blood sugar levels begin to drop. Correspondingly, so do insulin levels. This is a signal to the body to tap into its energy reserves. The next available source of energy is the glycogen stored in the liver. The body has enough glycogen reserves to last between 24 and 36 hours. In the first day of fasting, our body is fueled by glycogen.

Within 24 hours, the liver is becoming depleted of glycogen. The cells in the body still require fuel, so our bodies respond to the lack of available fuel by initiating a process known as *gluconeogenesis*. Gluconeogenesis means "new sugar creation." This is a process wherein glucose is manufactured from amino acids. For between 24 and 48 hours following your final meal, this is how your body fuels its metabolism.

Between 48 and 72 hours after your final meal, the body enters into a state of ketosis. Ketosis is a metabolic state wherein the body taps into its reserves of fat for fuel in lieu of glucose. At this point in the fast, prolonged levels of lowered insulin signal to the body to initiate *lipolysis*, which is the breakdown of triglycerides. *Triglycerides* are the form of fat used as energy storage.

Triglycerides are broken down into a glycerol backbone molecule, which is utilized for gluconeogenesis, and fatty acid molecules. The fatty acid molecules can be used as energy for most tissues in the body; the primary exception to this is the brain. The body responds by creating ketone bodies, which cross the blood-brain barrier and can be utilized by the brain as fuel.

Ninety-six hours into fasting, 75% of the brain's energy is derived from ketone bodies, primarily beta-hydroxybutyrate and acetoacetate. In a fasted state, these ketone bodies increase up to 70 times their normal levels. (1) The significant presence of these ketone bodies is what causes "keto breath." For some people in a state of ketosis, they might have a metallic taste in their mouth. It can have a fruity scent, or even smell like nail polish!

By 120 hours, basic metabolism is almost entirely supplied by fatty acids and ketone bodies. Blood sugar levels, however, do not drop below healthy levels; this is due to the fact that gluconeogenesis is now supplied by glycerol backbones made available by lipolysis.

During this phase of the fast, protein conservation is initiated in the body. Protein turnover remains normal, however, and no proteins are used for energy. (2) This is important, because one critique of fasting is that the process will essentially cannibalize lean muscle mass. This, however, is largely a myth. Certainly, in a state of starvation from prolonged malnutrition, this can happen, but when fasting is executed in the right way, your body does not "eat" your muscles for energy. Instead, your body primarily switches to lipolysis, or using its fat reserves for energy.

At around 120 hours into a fast, levels of norepinephrine and human growth hormone are also notably increased.

What we have largely described is the body switching from using glucose for fuel to stored fat, and while we are only five days into our fast, we know that people can (and have) fasted for longer periods of time. In chapter two, we discussed the case of a morbidly obese man who was observed to have fasted for well over a year with nothing but water and vitamin/mineral supplementation. The only effects were the resolution of his obesity.

Given enough fat reserves, and provided certain vitamins and minerals are supplemented, we do not know of a limit on how long a person can go without caloric consumption. All of this, of course, is within reason; certainly, for a person with minimal fat reserves, the line between fasting and starvation is much closer. Fasting is not starvation, and beyond the possibility of the health benefits conferred by fasting, no one should ever fast into a malnourished state.

Noteworthy Effects of Fasting

All of what I have described are the metabolic changes associated with fasting. Let's take a closer look at some of the health benefits associated with these metabolic changes to the body.

Lower Insulin Levels

As we discussed, insulin is an important hormone, as it both ushers glucose into cells for use as energy and assists us with storing excess glucose to be burned as energy later. Insulin is also used to usher nutrients, such as magnesium, into cells. Insulin, therefore, is very important for keeping our cells supplied with energy and nutrients—the things they need to carry out their lifecycle, maintain their energy levels, and remain healthy.

One of the biggest health problems facing the developed world, however, is that of insulin resistance, which is a sign of what's called *metabolic syndrome*. When you become insulin resistant, your cells become less sensitive to insulin, which prevents insulin from ushering glucose and other nutrients into your cells the way it normally would. Because your cells respond less efficiently to insulin, levels of glucose in the blood remain frequently elevated.

There are a number of health problems associated with metabolic syndrome, including insatiable appetite, increased weight that is difficult to lose, high triglycerides, high blood pressure, skin issues, and hormonal problems. If allowed to progress, insulin resistance eventually results in type 2 diabetes. These issues, however, are alarmingly common in the United States. In 2020, the CDC reported that 34 million Americans—a little more than 1 in 10—are diabetic, and 88 million Americans are pre-diabetic, or considered insulin resistant, which for many can progress into diabetes if left unmitigated. (4)

Type 2 diabetes is a horrible disease that brings the risk of a number of complications, including damage to the eyes and kidneys and amputation of limbs. Diabetes also increases the risk of developing other diseases, such as cardiovascular disease and Alzheimer's disease. And, for our discussion on cancer, diabetes is a risk factor that increases the likelihood of developing cancer—something we expand upon in the following chapter. (5)

This is one reason why the insulin-lowering abilities of fasting might be so beneficial. If you eat all the time, your body is responding by constantly raising insulin, which will rise as a result of eating carbohydrates or protein, particularly animal protein. Fasting is one of the best ways to lower insulin, and the longer the fast, the lower the levels of insulin.

Studies done in rats have demonstrated the ability of intermittent fasting (fasting for 16 hours a day while only eating in a window of 8 hours) to reverse insulin resistance, lower obesity, reduce systemic inflammation, and even reverse diabetes. Interestingly, some of these effects were observed independently of any sort of caloric restriction during the feeding window, meaning the beneficial effects on metabolic health were the direct result of fasting. (6, 7) Furthermore, there is evidence that these noteworthy effects of fasting extend to humans as well. (8)

Regularly lowering your insulin level not only improves insulin resistance—an important precursor to developing type 2 diabetes—but will help rid the body of excess water and salt and will help improve blood pressure levels. (1)

There are, of course, other ways to lower insulin levels; these include measures such as eating a diet low in refined carbohydrates, eating healthy amounts of fiber, and regularly exercising. The effects of fasting on insulin levels, however, are well documented and a key component of fasting's health benefits. When it comes to maintaining healthy insulin levels and preventing the insulin resistance that leads to diabetes, fasting is potentially a very important tool.

Increased Levels of Human Growth Hormone

Human growth hormone, or *HGH*, is produced by the pituitary gland and is what prompts our bodies to grow as adolescents. HGH is an important factor as we age too; HGH plays a number of roles in the body, including regulating body composition, contributing to bone and muscle growth, regulating body fluids, boosting the immune system, and assisting in sugar and fat metabolism. HGH is also a counter-regulatory hormone; when we are in a fasted state, HGH prevents the body from going into "starvation mode." Each morning before you wake up, you experience a surge of HGH which helps raise blood sugar levels, providing energy in a fasted state.

The production of HGH declines as we age. By the age of 40, our HGH production is cut by 30%, and by 60 it can decline as much as 80%. Lowered HGH in adults is associated with excess fat, lower lean muscle mass, and decreased bone density. HGH is included in a list of "miracle" anti-aging hormones, and many people use HGH as an anti-aging antidote. This is ill-advised, however, because exogenous (*exogenous means originates outside of the body*) HGH is known to raise blood sugar and blood pressure and is associated with an increased risk of certain cancers. (9)

Fasting, however, is known to increase levels of natural human growth hormone. Fasting as little as two days can elicit a 5X increase in HGH, while longer fasts can raise levels to as much as 12.5X. (1) This elevation of HGH is achieved without any of the negative side effects seen with the use of exogenous HGH. (10) In fact, we know that fasting can have *benefits* for both blood sugar levels and blood pressure levels.

Interestingly, eating a meal suppresses the secretion of HGH, so if we are eating throughout the day, we are not getting any HGH during the day at all. So while fasting increases our HGH—often dramatically—eating the way most people tend to eat, enjoying meals and snacks spread out throughout the day, works to suppress HGH. Similarly, very low-calorie diets can suppress levels of HGH. It seems as though fasting might be the best way to elevate HGH naturally without the negative side effects seen in hormone replacement therapies.

What are the benefits of elevated HGH? HGH signals the body to repair damaged cells, stimulates fat burning, supports lean muscle growth, keeps the bones strong, and keeps the immune system strong. HGH increases levels of lipoprotein and hepatic lipase, which are important for breaking down triglycerides and are also thought to stabilize blood sugar. HGH also helps maintain youthfulness in the skin. Elevating your HGH naturally through fasting might confer some important and elusive anti-aging benefits.

The increase in human growth hormone is also important from a metabolic perspective because the increase means you are not going to lose muscle mass as a result of fasting. Importantly, HGH puts your body in a state to build muscle and burn fat. This, too, helps dispel the myth that fasting will ruin muscle mass or tone; in fact, the very opposite might be true.

Two important questions we must consider are as follows: One, does growth hormone cause cancer? And two, does growth hormone from any source (including from fasting) cause the growth of cancer that already exists?

There have been many theories postulated about the relationship between growth hormone and cancer. On a simple level, if growth hormone were a significant cause of cancer, we would tend to see cancer predominate in those who have the highest levels of growth hormone. We know that adolescents have, by far, the highest amount of growth hormone circulating through their bodies. Conversely, elderly people have the lowest amount of growth hormone in their bodies. So if growth hormone were a major cause of cancer, we would tend to see it predominantly impacting children and adolescents, but we don't. Cancer is overwhelmingly a disease of aging, occurring during a time when growth hormone levels are very low.

We know that growth hormone can be used by cancer cells for fuel. This is, of course, also the case for glucose, amino acids, fats, cholesterol, iron, and some other hormones as well. After all, cancer cells are former normal cells that have mutated, so it makes sense that cancer cells use many of the same energy sources as healthy cells do.

However, we must ensure that we aren't inadvertently fueling cancer as a result of fasting. It turns out that although fasting temporarily increases growth hormone, it actually decreases insulin-like growth factor 1 (IGF1). IGF1 is a hormone that looks very similar to insulin and is stimulated by growth hormone. It is the IGF1 hormone that has been shown to promote cancer cell growth and spread while also stimulating angiogenesis. (11)

Fasting causes a reduction in IGF1 due to the action of a protein known as *insulin-like growth factor-binding protein 1* (*IGFBP1*). This IGFBP1 protein binds to IGF1 in the bloodstream and reduces the activity of IGF1. (12) So even though fasting temporarily increases growth hormone, it decreases IGF1 and thereby reduces a key fuel source that cancer wants to use.

Achieving Ketosis

It is worthwhile to take a moment to talk about the state of ketosis achieved by fasting. Many people are familiar with ketogenic diets, which have been popularized over the last few years. These diets have been touted by many for their many health benefits, including weight loss, and even their anti-cancer properties. However, many of the same benefits that can purportedly be derived from a ketogenic diet may also be derived from fasting.

A true, clinically noteworthy ketogenic diet is about 95% fat with some protein and virtually no carbohydrates; in practice, it is neither fun nor practical for people to follow. Knowing what we know about how fasting achieves lowered insulin levels and ultimately puts the body in a state of ketosis, it becomes obvious why keeping carbohydrates, and even protein, to an absolute minimum on a true ketogenic diet is necessary for achieving a state of ketosis.

Additionally, many people wind up eating lots of animal protein and high-fat dairy products while on a ketogenic diet. From a cancer perspective, this may not be the best way to eat, which is something we will discuss later on. Also, as I mentioned above, eating too much protein—particularly animal protein—still has the effect of raising insulin levels. Ultimately, fasting might be a better way to achieve some of the noteworthy effects associated with the ketogenic diet rather than following a diet that is difficult to truly follow from both a practical and clinical perspective and that is often followed in a way that is not always beneficial against cancer.

Fasting is perhaps the body's most natural way to achieve a state of ketosis. Ketosis, to reiterate, is the metabolic state wherein the body uses reserves of fat for energy instead of readily available glucose. Without the constant supply of protein and carbohydrates—and even dietary fats—the body must dip into its reserves of energy, which is stored fat.

Being in a state of ketosis has some profound health benefits. The most obvious benefit is that this is our body's way of burning fat reserves—the goal of anyone trying to lose weight. Fasting and ketosis are thought to have anti-inflammatory effects; this might be due to the fact that ketone metabolism creates less oxidative stress than glucose metabolism. A state of ketosis also has benefits for virtually every metabolic marker, including cholesterol levels, HbA1C, CRP, fasting insulin levels, blood sugar levels, and body fat. (13)

Being in a state of ketosis—particularly one facilitated by fasting—might have some very real benefits for our fight against cancer, which is covered in chapter 4. They key is getting into ketosis in a healthy way (via fasting, not a ketogenic diet) and not staying there too long.

Benefits for the Brain

Interestingly, fasting has shown some very real benefits for the health of our physical brain and our mental health. Some of these effects are likely due to being in a state of ketosis; 96 hours into fasting, 75% of the brain's energy is derived from ketone bodies, primarily beta-hydroxybutyrate (BHB) and acetoacetate. This is important because BHB is a more efficient source of energy for the brain than glucose; BHB provides more units of energy per unit of oxygen used. Ketones also inhibit the production of reactive oxygen species—oxidants—by up-regulating the activity of glutathione peroxidase, which is an important part of our body's natural antioxidant system. (14)

A 2018 study found some profound possible benefits for fasting and the brain, including the following:

- Improved cognition and sensory motor function
- Promotion of growth of new neurons and up-regulated neurotrophic factor
- Increased antioxidant protection of brain cells, lowering inflammation
- Stimulation of the growth of new mitochondria
- Promotion of autophagy of weak brain cells (15)

In addition to the physical benefits for our brains, there is evidence that the elevation of ketone bodies promoted by fasting might have anti-depressant and anti-anxiety effects. One study found that ketone bodies help regulate the nervous system through a receptor called GPR41; in a state of ketosis, there is a downregulation of the sympathetic nervous system and a slowing of heart rate.

Certainly, for people who are not used to fasting, beginning a fasting regimen can be tough; usually, the first few days can be uncomfortable. Anecdotal evidence suggests that many people who stick with a fasting regimen experience a lift of "brain fog" and increased mental clarity, in addition to invigorating energy. This is unsurprising, given what we know about the metabolic effects of fasting. We will cover more about how to implement fasting, including what to expect and how to overcome obstacles to getting started on a fasting regimen, in chapter 9.

Increased Metabolic Rate
Many people are opposed to trying fasting because it is falsely assumed that fasting will wreck your metabolism and you will feel tired, sluggish, and become unable to lose weight, etc. What we know about fasting is that when it is done appropriately, fasting actually *increases* your metabolic rate. (16)

Ironically, two of the strategies that have been most employed as a modality for weight loss and thus elevated health are two of the worst things for our metabolism. These include low-calorie diets and eating multiple meals throughout the day.

Prolonged low-calorie diets force our body to lower our baseline metabolic rate as it adapts to routinely being given insufficient energy. (13) The result is that many people have a difficult time losing weight, even though they are eating low-calorie diets. Eating throughout the day suppresses human growth hormone (1) and puts our bodies at a disadvantage metabolically to burn through stores of fat.

Two of the downstream effects of regular fasting, including a rise in HGH and the promotion of ketosis for energy, are both beneficial for metabolism. As HGH increases, your body is in a better position to build lean muscle and burn fat. HGH also prevents your body from going into starvation mode or cannibalizing muscle protein for energy.

Promotion of ketosis means the body is switching from using glucose exclusively as fuel, to fatty acids and ketones. The glycerol backbone makes gluconeogenesis possible, meaning blood sugar never dips to levels that would otherwise be dangerous.

Of course, these effects are only made possible when a proper amount of calories are consumed in feeding windows. Whatever type of fast you are participating in, it is important to get enough calories and nutrition when you do eat; we discuss how to eat in a way that best prevents cancer in chapter 6.

Fasting is also known to increase norepinephrine—adrenaline. (17) During periods of fasting, adrenaline is used to facilitate the release of stored glycogen and promote the burning of fat, thus stimulating the metabolism. Adrenaline also leaves those fasting with invigorated energy as opposed to feeling sluggish. In fact, many people who are in a fasted state report feeling increased energy and mental clarity.

In a four-day fasted state, resting energy expenditure was shown to have increased by 12% (17); in other words, fasting speeds up the metabolism as opposed to slowing it down.

Other Observations

One of the most fascinating things about fasting is that all of these effects are achieved through something completely natural, and at least in the context of human history, something that is totally normal, even if it is a state that has become abnormal to modern humans. The ability of the body to have mechanisms in place to deal with a fasted state is a testament to the fact that our bodies are clearly designed to deal with periods of not eating quite well; the fact that we are discovering so many associated benefits of fasting compels me to believe that fasting is not just a state we were designed to endure in emergencies, but a state our bodies *should* regularly endure.

One other noteworthy observation is a stunning lack of *negative* side effects associated with fasting in people with no other obvious contraindications.

Potential Side Effects of Fasting and How to Control Them

Fasting is not something many people in today's world are used to doing, so there are some things you should be aware of as you begin your fasting journey. By and large, when executed properly, fasting can be a very safe way to achieve many health benefits. Depending on how you choose to fast (something covered in chapter 9, "How to Fast"), there are different tools you can employ to prevent some of the potential negative side effects of fasting.

Dehydration is one of the most common side effects of fasting; this is obviously something we should seek to avoid. Some practitioners suggest that during your fast you should abstain from everything, including water, but in reality, there is absolutely no medical benefit to denying your body water, particularly during a fast. Getting enough water is critical for health. Virtually all of the chemical reactions in your body require the presence of water to take place. Staying hydrated is simply very important.

Furthermore, water has no calories and does not constitute breaking a fast. Drinking water does not cause a rise in insulin or blood sugar. Not only will drinking plenty of water during a fast not interfere with any of the benefits conferred by fasting, but it will also prevent some of the most common side effects from fasting. These include headache, dizziness, and fatigue—some of the most common side effects when you begin fasting.

When you are fasting, the drop in insulin means your body will shed excess fluid via urination. Combine this with the fact that at least a portion of our hydration comes not just from fluids but also from foods, and you can see why when you fast, it is actually much easier to become dehydrated.

The other thing your body sheds very quickly during a fast are electrolytes. These include nutrients like sodium (salt), potassium, and magnesium. Electrolytes are intimately linked with hydration, which is why they are included in sports drinks. Getting enough electrolytes helps you stay hydrated properly. When you are deficient in electrolytes, however, dehydration is only one of the potential side effects. Other side effects include muscle cramps and spasms, changes in heart rate, anxiety, problems sleeping, dizziness, fatigue, headaches, and low blood pressure.

When you are fasting, it may be beneficial to supplement with electrolytes. Adding things like salt, potassium chloride, and magnesium glycinate to water and drinking throughout the day can help ensure that you remain hydrated during a fast and do not deplete levels of electrolytes.

On the other hand, it is best to avoid any sort of sports drink, even the no-calorie varieties. These contain artificial sweeteners that may actually inadvertently raise your insulin levels and might cause an intensification of hunger. Even natural sources of electrolytes, like coconut water, should be avoided, as these contain calories that will break your fast. Water supplemented with electrolytes is the best way to maintain hydration and prevent many of the most common negative side effects associated with fasting.

Talk to your doctor before you begin to supplement with electrolytes, however, particularly if you have kidney problems or are on medications.

Constipation can be another challenge for those on a fast. Certainly, you would expect bowel movements to slow down when you are not eating, but if you are struggling with constipation, there are a few things you can do. First, be sure you are hydrated, because dehydration can cause constipation. During feeding times, be sure to consume enough fiber in the form of fruits, vegetables, and whole grains. We cover how you should eat during feeding times—particularly if you are using both diet and fasting as a modality against cancer—in later chapters.

Feeling cold can also be a side effect some people experience, particularly around the 24-hour period of your fast. This affects people differently and with varying degrees of intensity. Some people simply experience chilled extremities; some people get cold to the extent that they need to put more clothes on or turn on the heater. This is a normal response to fasting. Fasting is thought to stimulate the parasympathetic nervous system, promoting a state of relaxation and thus lowering blood pressure, heart rate, and body temperature. (13)

If this is something you experience during a fast, there are a few things you can do: Try getting some sunshine, take a warm shower, or simply layer up. As your body becomes more accustomed to fasting, these feelings will eventually dissipate.

•———————•

References:

(1) Fung, Jason, and Jimmy Moore. "What Is Fasting?" *The Complete Guide to Fasting: Heal Your Body through Intermittent, Alternate-Day, and Extended Fasting*, Victory Belt Publishing, Las Vegas, 2016.

(2) Nørrelund, Helene, et al. "Effects of GH on Protein Metabolism during Dietary Restriction in Man." *Growth Hormone & IGF Research*, vol. 12, no. 4, 2002, pp. 198–207., https://doi.org/10.1016/s1096-6374(02)00043-6.

(3) Khazan, Olga. "People Are Voluntarily Going Months without Food." *The Atlantic*, Atlantic Media Company, 16 June 2021, https://www.theatlantic.com/health/archive/2016/11/one-month-without-food/508220/.

(4) "National Diabetes Statistics Report." *Centers for Disease Control and Prevention*, Centers for Disease Control and Prevention, 7 Jan. 2022, https://www.cdc.gov/diabetes/library/features/diabetes-stat-report.html.

(5) Giovannucci, E., et al. "Diabetes and Cancer: A Consensus Report." *Diabetes Care*, vol. 33, no. 7, 2010, pp. 1674–1685., https://doi.org/10.2337/dc10-0666.

(6) Malaisse. "Intermittent Fasting Modulation of the Diabetic Syndrome in Sand Rats. II. in Vivo Investigations." *Interna-*

tional Journal of Molecular Medicine, vol. 26, no. 5, 2010, https://doi.org/10.3892/ijmm_00000523.

(7) Hatori, Megumi, et al. "Time-Restricted Feeding without Reducing Caloric Intake Prevents Metabolic Diseases in Mice Fed a High-Fat Diet." *Cell Metabolism*, vol. 15, no. 6, 2012, pp. 848–860., https://doi.org/10.1016/j.cmet.2012.04.019.

(8) Mattson, Mark P., et al. "Impact of Intermittent Fasting on Health and Disease Processes." *Ageing Research Reviews*, vol. 39, 2017, pp. 46–58. https://doi.org/10.1016/j.arr.2016.10.005.

(9) "Human Growth Hormone (HGH): Does It Slow Aging?" *Mayo Clinic*, Mayo Foundation for Medical Education and Research, 13 Nov. 2021, https://www.mayoclinic.org/healthy-lifestyle/healthy-aging/in-depth/growth-hormone/art-20045735.

(10) Ho, K. Y., et al. "Fasting Enhances Growth Hormone Secretion and Amplifies the Complex Rhythms of Growth Hormone Secretion in Man." *Journal of Clinical Investigation*, vol. 81, no. 4, 1988, pp. 968–975., https://doi.org/10.1172/jci113450.

(11) Jenkins P.J., Mukherjee A., Shalet S.M. "Does Growth Hormone Cause Cancer?" *Clin Endocrinol* (Oxf) 2006; 64(2): 115-21. doi: 10.1111/j.1365-2265.2005.02404.x.

(12) Brandhorst S., Choi I.Y., Wei M., et al. "A Periodic Diet that Mimics Fasting Promotes Multi-System Regeneration, Enhanced Cognitive Performance, and Healthspan." *Cell Metab* 2015; 22(1): 86-99. doi: 10.1016/j.cmet.2015.05.012.

(11) Jockers, David, and Michael Dugan. *The Fasting Transformation: A Functional Guide to Burn Fat, Heal Your Body and Transform Your Life with Intermittent & Extended Fasting*. DrJockers.com, 2020.

(12) Fan, Shelly. "The Fat-Fueled Brain: Unnatural or Advantageous?" *Scientific American Blog Network*, Scientific American, 1 Oct. 2013, https://blogs.scientificamerican.com/mind-guest-blog/the-fat-fueled-brain-unnatural-or-advantageous/#.

(13) Alirezaei, Mehrdad, et al. "Short-Term Fasting Induces Profound Neuronal Autophagy." *Autophagy*, vol. 6, no. 6, 2010, pp. 702–710., https://doi.org/10.4161/auto.6.6.12376.

(14) "Fasting Boosts Metabolism and Fights Aging." *Medical News Today*, MediLexicon International, https://www.medicalnewstoday.com/articles/324347.

(15) Zauner, Christian, et al. "Resting Energy Expenditure in Short-Term Starvation Is Increased as a Result of an Increase in Serum Norepinephrine." *The American Journal of Clinical Nutrition*, vol. 71, no. 6, 2000, pp. 1511–1515., https://doi.org/10.1093/ajcn/71.6.1511.

CHAPTER 4

Fasting and Cancer

What Science Says about the Relationship
Between Fasting and Cancer

It is quite clear that there are a myriad of benefits associated with fasting, and incorporating fasting into our lifestyles is a logical and relatively easy way to help avoid the serious health challenges that may await. (In chapter 9, we discuss how to incorporate fasting into your life.) And while there are many aspects of your health that can be potentially improved or rectified through fasting, we want to point our attention to one of the most profound benefits fasting may have to offer: very powerful anti-cancer effects.

The interest in fasting as a serious health- and longevity-promoting modality is still new, and similarly, there is still a lot of research to be done when it comes to our understanding of the ways fasting can both help prevent cancer and potentially aid in treatment. I am cautiously optimistic, because the current research points in a very positive direction: The downstream effects of integrating fasting into your routine seem to naturally put your body in a position to oppose cancer in some profound ways.

The Relationship Between Glucose, Insulin, And Cancer

Most people are aware of what insulin is, but it helps to refresh our minds about the vital role insulin plays in the body and why it is so crucial to our discussion on cancer.

Insulin is the hormone that helps our cells take in glucose. Glucose is simply a term for sugar in the blood. It is a simple form of sugar, one that our cells use to create energy, or ATP—the energy currency of our cells. The words *insulin* and *glucose* carry a negative connotation for some people, since the two terms are most commonly discussed when referring to diabetes. While it is certainly true that many people struggle to maintain healthy levels of both insulin and glucose in the body, and develop diabetes or pre-diabetes, the reality is that both insulin and glucose are necessary and vital parts of our body's metabolic system. The best way to think about insulin is that it helps your cells absorb glucose, which can then be used for energy to fuel the many metabolic processes in the body.

Foods such as bread, pasta, potatoes, or sweets are the most abundant source of simple carbohydrates, which are molecules that turn into glucose most readily during digestion. When you eat foods high in simple carbohydrates, your body receives signals to release insulin very quickly. In contrast, foods rich in complex carbohydrates and fiber take more time to digest into glucose, so the insulin surge is blunted by the more involved digestion process necessary to break down such foods. Examples of complex carbohydrates include vegetables, legumes, and whole grains. Similarly, foods rich in protein and fat are also ultimately broken down into glucose, but there are a greater number of steps necessary to achieve this outcome. As a result, the insulin spike resulting from consuming foods such as meat, eggs, olive oil, and nuts is also far less than eating simple carbohydrates. Remember, one of the primary goals of digestion is to break down the food we eat into its constituent components—carbohydrates into sugars, proteins into amino acids, and fats into fatty acids—so that these energy sources can be absorbed and used for fuel.

Over time, our cells can become resistant to the effects of insulin. More and more insulin is needed to usher the same amount of sugar into our cells. Insulin resistance makes our cells less capable of absorbing sugar to use as energy. Subsequently, levels of insulin and blood sugar remain high. Over time, you might begin to see your blood sugar levels creep up at your yearly physical. When our cells become too resistant to insulin, the levels of glucose in the blood remain perpetually high, and once fasting blood sugar consistently remains above a certain threshold, a person can be diagnosed with type 2 diabetes.

Type 2 diabetes is, of course, an enormous problem in the developed world, particularly in the United States. According to the CDC, in 2022 there were 28.7 million Americans diagnosed with diabetes, and there are as many as 8.5 million Americans living with undiagnosed diabetes. These numbers are staggering on their own, representing 11.3% of the population. (1) Diabetics have a heightened risk of many downstream problems, including blindness, limb amputation, kidney failure, stroke, and heart disease. Why this is important to our discussion, however, is that diabetics are at a much-heightened risk for developing cancer as well.

In 2018, researchers reviewed 47 studies from across the world. Led by Dr. Toshiaki Ohkuma from the George Institute for Global Health at the University of New South Wales in Sydney, Australia, the team—which included researchers from Oxford and Johns Hopkins Universities—concluded that women with diabetes were 27% more likely to develop cancer than women without diabetes, and men with diabetes were 19% more likely to develop cancer than men without diabetes. Dr. Ohkuma was quoted in the study as saying, "The link between diabetes and the risk of developing cancer is now firmly established." (5, 6)

The path to type 2 diabetes, however, is more like a gray-scale spectrum instead of a stark black-and-white image. In other words, you do not progress from being perfectly healthy to having diabetes overnight. Insulin resistance is the precursor to type 2 diabetes, also referred to as *pre-diabetes*. What we see in pre-diabetes is both insulin and blood sugar perpetually staying higher than they otherwise would be for prolonged periods of time. And according to the CDC, as many as 96 million Americans over the age of 18 are thought to have pre-diabetes—38% of the adult population! (1) These numbers are astounding, not only in terms of the potential scope of necessary medical care they portend, but also because pre-diabetics are also at an increased risk for developing cancer. (4)

These two groups of people—diabetes and pre-diabetics—represent over a third of the United States' population. The side effects of diabetes should be terrifying enough, but they become even more frightening when viewed in the context of increased cancer risk. The prevalence of diabetes and pre-diabetes certainly foreshadows a wave of potential cancer cases, and given the already enormous burden of cancer, the future can certainly look bleak in this regard. It shouldn't be surprising that the prevalence of cancer in the United States has increased along with the incidence of diabetes and pre-diabetes.

When we look at some of the metabolic properties of cancer, this relationship between diabetes, pre-diabetes, and cancer development comes into sharper focus. Cancer cells are highly reliant on insulin. Because cancer cells are metabolically very active, they need more energy in order to rapidly divide and grow at a faster rate than normal, healthy cells. This necessitates more insulin. In fact, cancer cells have between 15 and 16 times the number of insulin receptors as normal cells!

Someone who is diabetic or insulin resistant is going to have a lot more free insulin in their body than someone who is insulin sensitive. And certainly, if you already have cancer cells in your body and you are insulin resistant, all of that insulin floating around freely can be problematic.

Interestingly, some of the research done on diabetes medication provides some insight into the profound relationship between diabetes, pre-diabetes, and cancer. Metformin is a common drug given to diabetics. Studies have found that diabetics with no known cancer who were given metformin had a significantly lower risk of developing cancer than diabetics who were not given metformin. Additionally, the risk for cancer development for diabetics on metformin was *lower than non-diabetics.* (38, 39)

Metformin works by improving insulin sensitivity, thus reducing the need for so much insulin in the body and lowering blood sugar levels by improving insulin's efficacy. Metformin is something I use regularly in my clinic as repurposed medication for cancer treatment.

It is safe, well-tolerated, and cheap, and it is one of the most popular medications used off-label for cancer treatment.

Hyperglycemia and Cancer

Having chronically elevated levels of insulin is not the only mechanism in both diabetics and pre-diabetics that is implicated in the increased risk of cancer. Otto Warburg won the Nobel Prize in Medicine in 1931 for his discovery that cancer cells heavily rely on sugar for their energy synthesis. So we have known for some time that there is an intimate relationship between sugar and cancer. It is only in recent years, however, that the full scope of that relationship and its implications have come into focus. It turns out, cancer not only relies on glucose for energy, but prolonged, high levels of blood sugar, or hyperglycemia, might also play a role in facilitating cancer formation.

In 2019, a study conducted by City of Hope, a research center in California specializing in both cancer and diabetes, concluded that elevated levels of blood sugar can alter the structure of the DNA in our cells, resulting in damage. Furthermore, high glucose levels can suppress normal repair functions, resulting in genomic instability. (2) John Termini, PhD, a researcher at City of Hope, stated the following: "Genetic instability can cause and promote the progression of cancer . . . as the incidence of diabetes continues to rise, the cancer rates will likely increase as well." (3)

When we take into account the well-established link between cancer and diabetes/pre-diabetes, and the overwhelming scale at which these two conditions afflict people in our country, it is clear that intervening immediately is necessary to prevent the ongoing tidal wave of new cancer cases in the United States. Given the burden that cancer already represents, it is clear that we must take intentional steps to control factors such as insulin and glucose that facilitate cancer formation.

How Fasting Affects Insulin and Glucose Levels

The biggest factors implicated in the development of pre-diabetes and its progression into type 2 diabetes are poor diet and lack of exercise. Of course, we are accustomed to hearing this, because diet and exercise are the two biggest lifestyle factors that inform the health we do or do not experience.

Certainly, the standard American diet, a diet rich in processed foods that are high in unhealthy fats and simple carbohydrates while being void of fiber, nutrients, and protein, represents the ideal diet if you *want* to develop insulin resistance. And while a sedentary lifestyle is known to encourage insulin resistance, exercise is known to promote insulin sensitivity. (7) And while it is known that poor diet might facilitate insulin resistance, changing your diet can reverse insulin resistance and increase your sensitivity to insulin resistance. (8, 9)

While diet and exercise are key, fasting might prove to be as efficacious a strategy for lowering blood sugar and insulin levels. Theoretically, this makes sense. Remember, when you eat, your body is signaled to increase insulin production. When you are not eating, your body is not getting those same signals. Fasting gives insulin production a break. And when you are purposely *not* eating for a period of time, this allows your body to use existing blood sugar and tap into reserves of glycogen. Always keep in mind that your body is well-equipped to provide a steady supply of fuel to your cells, even in a fasted state. This is particularly true if you are carrying excess fat.

In this case, theory seems to be consistent with real-world results. A meta-analysis published in March of 2022 reviewed the effects of intermittent fasting on glucose/lipid metabolism and insulin resistance in patients with impaired glucose and lipid metabolism. What the authors found was that "intermittent fasting diets have certain therapeutic benefits on blood glucose and lipids in patients with metabolic syndrome (pre-diabetes) and significantly improve insulin resistance. (These) may be considered as an auxiliary treatment to prevent the occurrence and development of chronic disease." (10) So we can infer that if you are incorporating intermittent fasting into your regimen, you are not only helping control your blood sugar and insulin levels but are also reducing your risk of developing cancer.

Some of you might be thinking, "Yes, it makes sense that insulin and blood sugar levels drop when you are fasting. Can't the same results be achieved by eating a very low-carb diet, such as Atkins or a ketogenic diet?"

These types of diets are beneficial in lowering blood sugar and insulin levels, but the answer is more nuanced than that. The first thing to consider is that even diets higher in protein (especially animal protein), such as the Atkins diet, do still spike your insulin even though they are low in carbohydrates. But sources of animal protein are high in another growth factor for cancer that might be beneficial to avoid: methionine. Lowering our intake of methionine is a good idea if we want to avoid cancer, which means many of the high-protein and high-fat diets people use to lower insulin and blood sugar may not be ideal as a comprehensive anti-cancer strategy. We cover more on what to eat when you are not fasting in the following chapters, but suffice it to say, I would not recommend trying to achieve healthy levels of insulin and blood sugar by eating steak, bacon, and cheddar cheese all the time.

The good news is that fasting elicits many of the same insulin- and blood sugar–lowering effects that we find with these types of diets, and it may even achieve better results than very-low-carbohydrate diets. One study in 2015 found that low-carb diets lowered insulin levels compared to that seen with a standard diet, but fasting reduced those levels even further. (11)

Fasting seems to be one of the best modalities we have available for achieving and maintaining healthy blood sugar and insulin levels. Particularly if you fall into the category of pre-diabetic, intermittent fasting might be one of the easiest and safest ways to reverse insulin resistance and make yourself more insulin sensitive, particularly when combined with healthy diet and exercise. The downstream effect of this is you put yourself in a good position to defend against cancer.

Fasting and Weight Control

Maintaining a healthy weight is one of the most useful yet often disregarded strategies for fighting cancer. Carrying too much weight is associated with an increased risk of developing cancer. Carrying extra weight is thought to be responsible for 11% of cancers in women and 5% of cancers in men in the US, and 7% of cancer deaths overall. (12) I believe that the actual number is probably higher. In addition, it is worth noting that overweight cancer patients usually have a poorer prognosis than cancer patients who are at a healthy weight.

We as a society are overwhelmingly carrying too much weight. Obesity prevalence in the United States was 41.9% for adults age 20 in 2020 according to the CDC. (13) An additional 32.3% of people are considered overweight while not quite meeting the threshold to be considered obese. In total, people who are overweight or obese represent nearly three-quarters of the population in the United States, or 73.6% of people. All of these numbers are grim on their own, but the future looks even bleaker when we factor in the rate of childhood obesity, which has grown astronomically in recent years. We have a weight problem in the United States, and anything we can do to rectify that will help us fight cancer now and in the future.

Interestingly, being overweight is closely related to insulin resistance. People who are pre-diabetic often experience a cluster of health issues, including carrying excess weight (particularly around the waist), high blood sugar levels, high blood pressure, and irregular cholesterol and triglyceride levels. This is collectively often referred to as *metabolic disease*. Having metabolic disease also puts you at an increased risk of cancer. (14)

Metabolic disease, pre-diabetes, and even type 2 diabetes are all lifestyle diseases, meaning we develop them as a result of poor diet, lack of exercise, and other less-than-optimal lifestyle factors such as poor sleep and chronic stress. All of these conditions can pave the way for cancer formation, but often, one of the first signs that you are developing these diseases or are at risk of getting them is carrying excess weight.

Our bodies are designed to store fat, and there is no known limit to the amount of excess fat that can be stored in our bodies. But what was once a survival mechanism that helped our ancestors through times of famine has become a plague of modern society. Again, we can certainly implicate the diet most people eat, which is rich in processed foods comprised of sugar, simple carbohydrates, unhealthy fats, preservatives, and any other number of non-food additives. But something must be said about the volume and frequency with which we eat that necessarily plays a role too. We have all heard the stories of people who have lost weight while simply eating fast food and junk food yet staying in a caloric deficit. While this is ill-advised, it offers insight into the role volume, and I believe frequency, plays in weight gain.

This is further evidenced by the studies done on fasting as it relates to weight loss. Most of the research points to fasting being an excellent modality for weight loss. A Canadian study found that intermittent fasting resulted in between 0.8% and 13% reduction of baseline body weight and that weight loss occurred regardless of caloric intake. BMI decreased on average by 4.3%. The studies analyzed lasted from 2 to 12 weeks. (15)

Fasting's ability to facilitate weight loss is likely in part due to its ability to help the body achieve ketosis, a state in which fat stores are used for cellular energy as opposed to glucose. And while ketogenic and very-low-carb diets have also been shown to be beneficial for weight loss, a true ketogenic diet is difficult in practice, since it comprises over 80% fat. Most people on low-carb and ketogenic diets focus on foods like high-fat meats and cheeses, but evidence points to the fact these are definitely not the foods we should be focusing on to protect ourselves against cancer.

Fasting represents a way to achieve these same results—ketosis and the subsequent associated weight loss—without relying primarily on animal products for nourishment or eating an extremely restricted diet. And while it does matter what you eat when you are not fasting, it is possible to focus on a wider spectrum of nourishing foods—even enjoying them in abundance—and still lose weight while committed to a fasting regimen.

I should offer one caveat here, which is that fasting does not necessarily need to be used to lose weight. Particularly in cancer patients, we do not want certain patients to lose too much weight or to experience wasting syndrome. That being said, fasting has benefits beyond just weight loss and might even have some benefits for cancer treatment.

Autophagy

One of the benefits of fasting is that it stimulates autophagy. *Autophagy* is a process wherein the waste products and damaged parts of our cells that accumulate therein as part of their natural processes are recycled. This is a beneficial process, as it reduces stress on our cells, helping to keep our cells healthy and stable.

Autophagy's relationship to cancer is profound. Think back to our analogy of the toxic bucket. Our cells can withstand a certain amount of toxic bombardment before they become too weak or damaged to carry out their cellular processes—every "hit" to our cells amounts to a splash in the bucket. When that bucket becomes too full, cellular DNA is damaged or mutates, and the cell becomes cancerous.

Autophagy represents one way of "emptying" that toxic bucket before it becomes too full. One study on the relationship between autophagy and cancer states the following:

> [Autophagy] is a conserved lysosomal degradation pathway for the intracellular recycling of macromolecules and clearance of damaged organelles and mis-folded proteins to ensure cellular homeostasis. Dysfunctional autophagy contributes to many diseases, including cancer. (17)

Another study on autophagy states the following:

> This . . . intracellular recycling provided by autophagy serves to maintain cellular homeostasis by eliminating superfluous or damaged proteins and organelles . . . Thus, autophagy promotes the health of cells . . . deregulation of autophagy is linked to susceptibility for various disorders including degenerative diseases, metabolic syndrome, aging, infectious diseases, and cancer . . . As a cytoprotective survival pathway, autophagy prevents chronic tissue damage and cell death that lead to cancer initiation and progression. As such, stimulation or restoration of autophagy may prevent cancer. (18)

In layman's terms, autophagy is a cellular renewal that can help prevent the cascade of processes in the cell that ultimately result in cancer. This is an important mechanism in the body and one we should seek to facilitate.

So when does autophagy take place? Most autophagy actually occurs when we are asleep! Coincidentally, autophagy occurs when you are fasting. However, if you are someone who eats right before bed, introducing a load of calories into your digestive tract, you will not experience autophagy. (19) Since autophagy occurs in a fasted state, it should come as no surprise that extending the fasted state is a great way to stimulate autophagy to a meaningful degree.

When we have heightened levels of glucose, insulin, and proteins, autophagy is turned off. When we eat carbohydrates or protein, heightened levels of insulin activate the mammalian target of rapamycin (mTOR) growth pathway. The body senses that there is plenty of energy, no cellular recycling is necessary, and autophagy is down-regulated in the body. This means that if you are someone who eats all day, you are constantly suppressing autophagy in your body.

When mTOR is dormant or unstimulated—such as in a fasted state—autophagy is switched back on. During this time, the worn-out parts of cells and cellular waste are recycled and sent back to the liver to be used to create energy (via gluconeogenesis) or to create new proteins to repair parts of the body. Our bodies are very efficient machines when we treat them properly! This process happens regardless of whether we have stored body fat or glycogen in the liver—it is merely stimulated by acute absences of nutrients, i.e., going periods without eating. (19)

The mTOR pathway plays a very important role in cancer progression. It has been established that mTOR is an important player in cancer cell growth, spread, and survival. (20) If we can disrupt the mTOR pathway, we stand a much greater chance of slowing cancer down. Interestingly, this is where the drug metformin comes in again. One of the mechanisms by which metformin is thought to fight cancer is by inhibiting the mTOR pathway. This is likely among the many reasons why it works well against cancer, including its ability to lower glucose and insulin levels. (21) Metformin inhibits this pathway, allowing for the process of autophagy to resume.

Fasting is one of the only known ways to inhibit the mTOR pathway without the use of drugs. Autophagy is thought to be stimulated between the 16-to-24-hour mark of fasting. So if you are engaging in intermittent fasting, such as a 16:8 fasting/feeding window, a 20:4

fasting/feeding window, or the OMAD (one meal a day) approach, you are stimulating this process in your body.

Extended fasts, however, might be a good way to stimulate this process even further. The longer into an extended fast, the more autophagy is stimulated. Autophagy is thought to peak at approximately day four on a fast. This is why some leading researchers, such as Dr. Thomas Seyfried, recommend participating in a once-per-year extended fast of up to a week to help prevent cancer. You can think of this as a "cellular cleanse."

Extended fasts are better suited for those experienced with fasting, but this idea of fasting for an extended period of time between three and seven days is not irregular in the context of history. Our ancestors necessarily would have endured periods of fasting which might have extended well beyond a week when food was scarce. While most people in the developed world do not go more than a day without eating, we see many of these beneficial biological processes being up-regulated by these slightly extended periods of going without food. Needless to say, there are risks associated with extended fasts, and I recommend that you speak with your doctor before trying an extended fast. But these types of fasts might have some real benefit for cancer prevention as well as cancer treatment, and it is very likely due in no small part to the stimulation of autophagy.

It is important to note that mTOR is not all bad. The mTOR growth pathway is important for the growth of healthy cells, including muscle cells. If we keep mTOR low all the time, we will be frail and unhealthy, preventing our normal cells from working optimally. So we do not want to reduce mTOR all the time. As with most things, it's all about balance. We want mTOR to be stimulated at the right times, such as during and after a workout, because it is beneficial to us. But we do not want to have mTOR turned on all the time, because having our bodies in a continuous growth state creates a cancer-promoting environment.

Other Factors Related to Cancer that Are Affected by Fasting

Fasting certainly seems to initiate a cascade of beneficial biological processes in the body, and in addition to some of the major benefits we have discussed above, there are other factors fasting facilitates that might have anti-cancer benefits.

Fasting Is Anti-Inflammatory

Fasting has the ability to help lower inflammation within the body. When we talk about the toxic environment that we can bathe our cells in—a process that helps fill up our so-called toxic bucket—part of what we are talking about is the chronic inflammation that engulfs many of the tissues in our bodies. This can be facilitated by many things, but lifestyle factors such as diet are among the triggers which can promote this chronic inflammation within the body.

Fasting can help lower this inflammation. One study on participants in Ramadan fasting found a reduction in pro-inflammatory cytokine concentrations. (22) We know that elevated inflammatory cytokines are implicated in cancer. (23)

Fasting also allows for better management of inflammatory cytokines interleukin-6 (IL-6) and tumor necrosis factor alpha (TNF-α), both of which are often elevated in cancer patients. (24, 25, 26) Fasting also lowers interleukin-8 (IL-8) signaling. IL-8 is an inflammatory molecule that is elevated when tumors are present and is thought to promote cell division, angiogenesis, and metastasis. (27, 28)

Fasting Stimulates Growth Hormone
The release of growth hormone is facilitated by sleep, but fasting is one way we can naturally boost growth hormone. Growth hormone serves a number of purposes, including burning fat, retaining muscle mass, and repairing damaged cells. Growth hormone might also be able to assist in DNA repair. (29)

Fasting Up-Regulates AMP-K
Fasting has been shown to up-regulate AMP-K, or adenosine monophosphate. (30, 31) AMP-K is a byproduct of ATP (adenosine triphosphate), or the energy currency of a cell. When the ratio of AMP is elevated in relation to ATP, this signals that energy is low in the cell. Up-regulating AMP-K is thought to divert glucose from cancer cells to healthy cells, (32) and potentially reverse metabolic damage in cancer cells. (33) It is worth noting that metformin also stimulates AMP-K.

Fasting Stimulates Apoptosis of Unhealthy Cells
We have discussed at length the process of autophagy, wherein cells recycle their damaged parts and waste products and use them as fuel. Equally as important as autophagy is the process of *apoptosis*, or *programmed cell death*.

Apoptosis sounds like something we should wish to avoid, but it is actually a healthy, normal, and very beneficial process. One of the problems with cancer cells is that they are immortal—they have no programmed death. On the contrary, healthy cells do have a programmed death. When our cells get worn out, they are supposed to die since they have fulfilled their purpose and can be replaced by younger, healthier cells.

One recent study noted that fasting between 24 and 72 hours facilitates cancer cell death. The speculation is that as the body switches from glucose to ketone bodies and oxidative phosphorylation for fuel, cancer cells (which, again, primarily rely on glucose for fuel) quickly die without a source of energy. The authors noted that fasting might make cancer cells more vulnerable to chemotherapy as well. (34)

Fasting and Cancer Treatment

Fasting has utility beyond just cancer prevention. In my clinic, we use fasting as a modality for cancer treatment. Indeed, fasting can work to both enhance the effects of chemotherapy and mitigate some of the harms associated with it.

While I do my best to integrate the best natural and alternative therapies into my practice, I do still use chemotherapy. For many, even the word *chemotherapy* has a negative, emotionally charged connotation, but the way we use chemotherapy in my clinic is quite different from how most clinics use it.

I use what is known as *fractionated metronomic chemotherapy*. If you go to a conventional oncology clinic, they will use your height and weight to calculate your maximum tolerated dosage of chemotherapy. You will be administered this dose every one to three weeks on average, depending on the chemotherapy agents used. Not surprisingly, when patients are given such a large dose of chemotherapy, significant side effects can—and often do—occur. In terms of the cancer itself, the main problem with this method of chemotherapy dosing and administration is the long window between treatments. This gap in therapy allows cancer time to mutate and become resistant to treatment in the future. This is why patients receiving conventional chemotherapy sometimes initially see a sharp reduction in their cancer, only to have the disease come roaring back later, stronger than ever.

In contrast, with fractionated metronomic chemotherapy, we calculate the maximum tolerated dosage in the same way, but we only administer 10–20% of that dosage, albeit more frequently. This gives cancer less time to mutate, and the side effects are greatly diminished, if not non-existent. We administer this dose three days per week.

To maximize the efficacy of fractionated chemotherapy, we take advantage of some of cancer's metabolic vulnerability. I have all of my patients fast prior to chemotherapy, at least 10–12 hours leading up to treatment. This helps prime cancer cells for the assault of chemotherapy heading their way.

In addition, just prior to chemotherapy being administered, we administer insulin and dextrose through a process known as *insulin potentiation therapy* (*IPT*). You can think of IPT as a delivery system to help chemotherapy work better. The insulin is used to activate as many cancer cells as possible at the time of treatment, while the dextrose (a form of sugar) is used to buffer the insulin to prevent blood sugar from becoming low.

We use IPT because we know that active cancer cells are vulnerable to chemotherapy, but dormant cancer cells are not. At any given time, a large subset of cancer cells is in the dormant state unless we do something to activate them. We are taking advantage of the fact that cancer cells have significantly more insulin and glucose receptors on their surface, and activating them using insulin potentiation therapy.

In essence, we are activating cancer cells under our supervision, at the time of treatment.

Chemotherapy given without attempting to increase the number of vulnerable cancer cells is a very inefficient process, especially when maximum tolerated dosing of chemotherapy is employed. The result is a blast of chemotherapy that has the potential to cause significant side effects while killing far fewer cancer cells than it could (since many potentially active cancer cells remain dormant).

As with many areas in oncology which fall outside the standard of care, we have good scientific support for IPT, but we do not have conclusive studies which would allow it to be incorporated into the current standard of care in traditional oncology practices. However, I can tell you that I see it work very well in my practice. I have found it to be very effective and also quite safe and well-tolerated.

In addition to using fasting as a complement to chemotherapy and IPT, there are other benefits as well. Some researchers have studied what fasting can do to enhance the effects of chemotherapy, and there have been at least three studies into the effects of fasting on chemotherapy regimens.

The first study in 2009 found that in 10 patients undergoing high-dose chemotherapy, fasting was found to lessen side effects, including fatigue, weakness, and digestive issues *without* lessening the effect the chemotherapy had on cancer. The fasting windows ranged from 48–140 hours leading up to treatment and 5–56 hours post-treatment. (35)

A 2016 study divided 20 patients into three groups. The first group fasted for 24 hours prior to chemotherapy; the second group fasted or 48 hours prior to chemotherapy.; and the third group fasted for 24 hours leading up to treatment and continued fasting for 48 hours after treatment. Lower levels of DNA damage and less inflammation were observed post-treatment in all three groups. While all patients experienced a reduction of symptoms, the longer fasting windows were most efficacious. (36)

Another study in 2018 used a 36-hour pre-treatment/24-hour post-treatment fasting window. Again, patients experienced a reduction in side effects associated with treatment. (37)

As a physician, I do believe that these lengthy fasting windows are a big ask for patients. A fast lasting 2, 3, or 4 days is difficult for many people to execute, particularly if you are not accustomed to fasting. Plus, dealing with cancer while going through cancer treatment, where fatigue and weakness are quite common, makes a multi-day fast nearly impossible. For these reasons, I have found a 10–12 hour fast, with a maximum of 16–18 hours of fasting, to work best for most cancer patients. This allows for the benefits of fasting while avoiding many of the pitfalls associated with longer-term fasts in the setting of cancer and cancer treatment.

Regardless of the fasting method chosen, it is undeniable that fasting is a beneficial modality for cancer treatment. As always, I encourage you to speak with your doctor before beginning a fast, especially if you have cancer and are receiving chemotherapy. It is also important to remember that fasting might affect other medicines you may be taking, so exercise caution.

References

(1) Centers for Disease Control and Prevention. (2022, January 18). *National Diabetes Statistics Report.* Centers for Disease Control and Prevention. Retrieved July 26, 2022, from https://www.cdc.gov/diabetes/data/statistics-report/index.html?ACSTrackingID=DM72996&ACSTrackingLabel=New+Report+Shares+Latest+Diabetes+Stats+&deliveryName=DM72996.

(2) Helwick, C. (n.d.). *Diabetes and Cancer: Researchers Link Hyperglycemia to DNA Damage.* The ASCO Post. Retrieved August 2, 2022, from https://ascopost.com/issues/october-10-2019/researchers-link-hyperglycemia-to-dna-damage/.

(3) *Diabetes Symptoms Could Cause Genomic Instability and Lead to Cancer.* City of Hope. (2022, May 11). Retrieved August 2, 2022, from https://www.cityofhope.org/news/diabetes-patients-and-increased-cancer-risk.

(4) Huang, Y., Cai, X., Qiu, M., Chen, P., Tang, H., Hu, Y., & Huang, Y. (2014). Prediabetes and the Risk of Cancer: A Meta-Analysis. *Diabetologia, 57*(11), 2261–2269. https://doi.org/10.1007/s00125-014-3361-2.

(5) MediLexicon International. (n.d.). "Link between diabetes and cancer risk firmly established." Medical News Today. Retrieved August 2, 2022, from https://www.medicalnewstoday.com/articles/322517#Women-at-higher-risk-than-men.

(6) "Cancer and Diabetes: The Connection Is in Your DNA." Cancer Treatment Centers of America. (2022, May 25). Retrieved August 2, 2022, from https://www.cancercenter.com/community/blog/2021/05/diabetes-cancer#:~:text=The%20

hormone%20insulin%20used%20to,another%20risk%20factor%20for%20cancer.

(7) Bollinger, L., & LaFontaine, T. (2011). Exercise Programming for Insulin Resistance. *Strength & Conditioning Journal, 33*(5), 44–47. https://doi.org/10.1519/ssc.0b013e31822599fb.

(8) Mirabelli, M., Russo, D., & Brunetti, A. (2020). "The Role of Diet on Insulin Sensitivity." *Nutrients, 12*(10), 3042. https://doi.org/10.3390/nu12103042.

(9) "Insulin Resistance: What It Is, Causes, Symptoms & Treatment." Cleveland Clinic. (n.d.). Retrieved August 2, 2022, from https://my.clevelandclinic.org/health/diseases/22206-insulin-resistance.

(10) Yuan, X., Wang, J., Yang, S., Gao, M., Cao, L., Li, X., Hong, D., Tian, S., & Sun, C. (2022). "Effect of Intermittent Fasting Diet on Glucose and Lipid Metabolism and Insulin Resistance in Patients with Impaired Glucose and Lipid Metabolism: A Systematic Review and Meta-Analysis." *International Journal of Endocrinology, 2022*, 1–9. https://doi.org/10.1155/2022/6999907.

(11) Frank Q. Nuttall, Rami A. Almokayyad, and Mary C. Gannon, "Comparison of a Carbohydrate-Free Diet Vs. Fasting on Plasma Glucose, Insulin and Glucagon in Type 2 Diabetes," *Metabolism: Clinical and Experimental* 64, vol. 2 (2015): 253-62.

(12) "Does Body Weight Affect Cancer Risk?" American Cancer Society. (n.d.). Retrieved August 3, 2022, from https://www.cancer.org/healthy/cancer-causes/diet-physical-activity/body-weight-and-cancer-risk/effects.html.

(13) "Diabetes Symptoms Could Cause Genomic Instability and Lead to Cancer." City of Hope. (2022, May 11). Retrieved August 2, 2022, from https://www.cityofhope.org/news/diabetes-patients-and-increased-cancer-risk.

(14) M. D. Anderson Cancer Center, & Underferth, D. (2021, June 17). "What Is Metabolic Syndrome?" M. D. Anderson Cancer Center. Retrieved August 3, 2022, from https://www.mdanderson.org/cancerwise/what-is-metabolic-syndrome.h00-159461634.html.

(15) Welton S., Minty R., O'Driscoll T., Willms H., Poirier D., Madden S., Kelly L. "Intermittent Fasting and Weight Loss: Systematic Review." *Can Fam Physician*. 2020 Feb;66(2):117-125. PMID: 32060194; PMCID: PMC7021351.

(16) Centers for Disease Control and Prevention. (2022, April 20). "FastStats - Overweight Prevalence." Centers for Disease Control and Prevention. Retrieved August 3, 2022, from https://www.cdc.gov/nchs/fastats/obesity-overweight.htm.

(17) Antunes F., Erustes A.G., Costa A.J., Nascimento A.C., Bincoletto C., Ureshino R.P., Pereira G.J.S., Smaili S.S. "Autophagy and Intermittent Fasting: The Connection For Cancer Therapy?" *Clinics* (Sao Paulo). 2018 Dec 10;73(suppl 1):e814s. doi: 10.6061/clinics/2018/e814s. PMID: 30540126; PMCID: PMC6257056.

(18) "Autophagy: Recycling Is Good For Your Body Too." Cedars. (n.d.). Retrieved August 3, 2022, from https://www.cedars-sinai.org/blog/autophagy.html.

(19) Fung, J., & Moore, J. (2016). *The Complete Guide to Fasting: Heal Your Body Through Intermittent, Alternate-Day, and Extended Fasting.* Victory Belt Publishing.

(20) Chiang G.G., Abraham R.T. "Targeting the mTOR Signaling Network in Cancer." *Trends Mol Med* 2007; 13: 433-442.

(21) Guertin D.A., Sabatini D.M. "Defining the Role of mTOR in Cancer." *Cancer Cell* 2007 Jul; 12(1): 9-22.

(22) Faris M.A., et al. "Intermittent Fasting During Ramadan Attenuates Pro-inflammatory Cytokines an Immune Cells in Healthy Subjects." *Nutrition Research*, Vol. 32, No. 12, Dec 2012.

(23) Spranger J., et al. "Inflammatory Cytokines and the Risk to Develop Type 2 Diabetes: Results of the Prospective Population-Based European Prospective Investigation into Cancer and Nutrition (EPI Potsdam Study)." *Diabetes*, Vol. 52, No. 3, Mar 2003.

(24) Faris M.A., Kacimi S., Al-Kurd R.A., Fararjeh M.A., Bustanji Y.K., Mohammad M.K., Sale M.L. "Intermittent Fasting During Ramadan Attenuates Proinflammatory Cytokines and Immune Cells in Healthy Subjects." *Nutr Res.* 2012 Dec;32(12):947-55. PMID: 23244540.

(25) Vasconcelos A.R., Yshii L.M., Viel T.A., et al. "Intermittent Fasting Attenuates Lipopolysaccharide-Induced Neuroinflammation and Memory Impairment." *Journal of Neuroinflammation.* 2-14;11:85.

(26) Aksungar F.B., Topkaya A.E., Akyildiz M. "Interleukin-6, C-Reactive Protein and Biochemical Parameters During Prolonged Intermittent Fasting." *Ann Nutr Metab.* PMID: 17374948.

(27) Waugh D.J., Wilson C. The Interleukin-8 Pathway in Cancer." *Clin Cancer Res.* 2008;14(21):6735-41. PMID: 18980965.

(28) Unalacak M., Kara I.H., Baltaci D., Erdem O., Bucaktepe P.G. "Effects of Ramadan Fasting on Biochemical and Hematological Parameters and Cytokines in Healthy and Obese Individuals." *Metab Syndr Relat Disord.* 2011;9(2):157-61. PMID: 21235381.

(29) Jockers, D., & Dugan, M. (2020). "The Fasting Transformation: A Functional Guide to Burn Fat, Heal Your Body and Transform Your Life with Intermittent & Extended Fasting." DrJockers.com.

(30) Draznin, B., Wang, C., Adochio, R., Leitner, J. W., & Cornier, M. A. (2012). "Effect of Dietary Macronutrient Composition on AMP and SIRT1 Expression and Activity in Human Skeletal Muscle." *Hormone and Metabolic Research*, 44(9), 650-655. PMID:22674476.

(31) Cantó, C., Jiang, L. Q., Deshmukh, A. S., Mataki, C., Coste, A., Lagouge, M., Auwerx, J. (2010). "Interdependence of AMPK and SIRT1 for Metabolic Adaptation to Fasting and Exercise in Skeletal Muscle." *Cell Metabolism*, 11(3), 213-219. PMID: 20197054.

(32) Shackelford, D. B., & Shaw, R. J. (2009). "The LKB1-AMPK Pathway: Metabolism and Growth Control in Tumour Suppression." *Nature Reviews Cancer*, 9(8), 563-575. PMID: 19629071.

(33) Faubert, B., Boily, G., Izreig, S., Griss, T., Samborska, B., Dong, Z., Jones, R. G. (2013). "AMPK Is a Negative Regulator of the Warburg Effect and Suppresses Tumor Growth in Vivo." *Cell Metabolism*, 17(1), 113-124. PMID:23274086.

(34) DeGroot S., Pijl H., Van der Hoeven J.J.M., Kroep J.R. "Effects of Short-Term Fasting on Cancer Treatment." *J Exp Clin Cancer Res.* 2019;38(1):209.

(35) Safdie F.M., Dorff T., Quinn D., et al. "Fasting and Cancer Treatment in Humans: A Case Series Report." *Aging* (Albany NY). 2009;1(12):988-1007.

(36) Dorff T.B., Groshen S., Garcia A., et al. "Safety and Feasibility of Fasting in Combination with Platinum-Based Chemotherapy." *BMC Cancer.* 2016;16:360.

(37) Bauersfeld S.P., Kessler C.S., Wischnewsky M., et al. "The Effects of Short-Term Fasting on Quality of Life and Tolerance to Chemotherapy in Patients with Breast and Ovarian Cancer: A Randomized Cross-Over Pilot Study." *BMC Cancer.* 2018;18(1):476.

(38) Gandini S., Puntoni M., Heckman-Stoddard B.M., et al. "Metformin and Cancer Risk and Mortality: A Systematic Review and Meta-Analysis Taking into Account Biases and Confounders." *Cancer Prev Res (Phila)* 2014; 7(9): 867-85. doi: 10.1158/1940-6207.

(39) Decensi A., Puntoni M., Goodwin P., et al. "Metformin and Cancer Risk in Diabetic Patients: A Systematic Review and Meta-Analysis." *Cancer Prev Res (Phila)* 2010; 3(11): 1451-61. doi: 10.1158/1940-6207.

CHAPTER 5

What about When I'm Not Fasting? The Role of Diet

While we have discussed the role that fasting plays in health and in cancer, the other side of that discussion must include what you do when you are not fasting: eating. Likely, as far "natural" or "alternative" treatments for cancer go, the role that diet plays in cancer prevention and treatment has garnered some of the most interest . . . and speculation.

Cancer: The Benefits and Shortcomings of Dietary Recommendations

Arguably, there is no more fundamental factor that informs the health you do or do not experience than what you eat. The saying, "You are what you eat," describes some very literal truth. Food is our body's fuel and building material, and similar to how it matters what you put into your gas tank or what materials you use to construct a building, what we consume does matter.

Diet has been linked to some of the more serious diseases people experience, including but not limited to heart disease, diabetes, and, yes, cancer. Fortunately, for heart disease and diabetes, there are official dietary recommendations promoted by the medical community with the aim of preventing these diseases. The messaging around these diseases as far as dietary factors and other lifestyle factors has been exceedingly clear and well-promoted, to the extent that the general public has some idea about the role diet can play in these diseases. This subsequently allows individuals to make informed decisions about what they should and should not eat. The same cannot be said for cancer.

Part of the problem with the messaging surrounding cancer from the medical establishment is that cancer is still promoted as a genetic disease. Yet, a case can be made (which I did make in chapter 1) that thinking of cancer purely as a genetic disease might be flawed, and that viewing cancer as a genetic disease precludes many of the upstream factors that illicit the genetic changes seen in cancer. Some research points toward the fact that only about 6–8% of cancer cases are purely genetic in origin. (1) This means the overwhelming majority of cancers are caused by other factors, including lifestyle factors such as nutrition.

However, the most common advice given when it comes to cancer prevention is to not smoke. While this is excellent advice, it is far from being complete. The reality is that there is very little official dietary advice promoted by the medical community when it comes to cancer. This, however, is in spite of the fact that there is a mounting body of evidence saying that lifestyle factors, particularly diet, can play a significant role in cancer prevention. In fact, it is estimated that as many as 40–50% of cancer cases could be avoided simply by changing some lifestyle factors, including diet. (2) Furthermore, we know from some smaller studies that cancer patients who eat better tend to have better outcomes in terms of treatment as well as mitigation of side effects. (3)

So we can reasonably conclude that, yes, nutrition does play a factor in cancer prevention, and it can be of some significant assistance to those undergoing cancer treatment as well. So what is preventing the medical community from taking a unilateral stance on the issue and promoting nutrition as a significant and effective modality against cancer?

While it is certainly time to change our messaging around diet and cancer, there are likely a number of reasons why the medical community has been slow to consistently promulgate any dietary recommendations.

Among the most important reasons is likely the vortex of misinformation surrounding diet's relationship to cancer. Just a cursory search of the internet can reveal an overwhelming amount of information on diet's role in cancer, and the vast majority of it is likely not particularly helpful. If you or a loved one has dealt with cancer, you have probably received unsolicited opinions from loved ones about various diets and programs, complete with advice about what you should and should not eat. This cascade of information is overwhelming to most people. To further complicate matters, most people lack the scientific background that oncologists posses that would allow them to accurately sift through this information, separate fact from fiction, and ultimately draw accurate conclusions. The truth is, when it comes to diet's role in cancer, many of the recommendations you find on the internet are based on very preliminary or flimsy science, and some of the information available on how diet affects cancer has no scientific validity whatsoever.

Realistically, you cannot cure your cancer with diet alone, as much as people would like to believe the opposite. The scientific literature confirms that people who exclusively use alternative methods of treating cancer, including a sole dependency on nutrition, have far poorer outcomes than those who do not. (4) Changing your diet, regardless of how you do it, is very unlikely to cure your cancer. Doing so is akin to relying on winning the lottery in order to become rich. It could happen, but it's a really bad strategy, and it's almost certainly not going to be successful.

The other uncomfortable truth is that, in addition to being unable to cure you of cancer, changing your diet is unlikely to *completely* protect you from ever developing cancer. Is diet useful toward this end? Absolutely! But unfortunately, nutrition is not a panacea. Even by our most optimistic estimates, dietary measures alone are not enough to prevent 100% of cancer diagnoses.

There are a few reasons why we know this. We know that cancer has existed in humans as long as we have been here—even in ancient times when diets were arguably "cleaner," or at least void of the many foods or food additives that are so often blamed for causing cancer. The other reason, as we have discussed, is that there are too many other factors independent of diet that can create environments in our cells that would eventually lead them to become cancerous; there is a cascade of factors and carcinogens that can fill our metaphorical toxic bucket, causing it to overflow. Diet is simply one of these factors, and even if you do change that one factor, it is simply not enough to guarantee you will never develop cancer.

So to recap, is nutrition important? Yes.

Is good nutrition likely to cure your cancer or even prevent cancer altogether? No.

Is nutrition still a powerful tool that we can use to our advantage against cancer? Yes!

When we combine what we eat with the advantages afforded us by when we eat and how much/how often we eat (fasting), diet is something we should all be focusing on when we are trying to cultivate a healthy lifestyle. So as we move forward, we do so with a pragmatic, science-based paradigm about the role nutrition can play in our fight against cancer.

Relearning How to Eat

It is no secret that the typical American's diet is fairly abysmal. If it were not, it is unlikely that we would be suffering from an epidemic of obesity, heart disease, diabetes, and cancer in this country. Many people rely heavily on fast food, take-out, or convenience store fare—most of which are foods that hardly resemble anything found in nature. Subsequently, it almost goes without saying that anything resembling that of most Americans' diets is not the best way to eat if we are to fight cancer. Collectively, it is time that we relearn how to eat.

A simple place to start is to eat "close to the earth." Eating close to the earth means eating foods found in nature, in their most whole and unprocessed (or minimally processed) form. Foods such as fruits, vegetables, grains, beans, nuts, and seeds should be our focus. Michael Pollan, author of *In Defense of Food: An Eater's Manifesto*, said it well: "Eat food. Not too much. Mostly plants."

I recommend a plant-heavy diet to my patients. The research firmly points toward the fact that plant foods are not only safe to eat and rich in nutrition, but they also confer anti-cancer benefits. However, I stop short of recommending a vegan diet for two reasons.

First, the term *vegan* has become an emotionally and politically charged term that understandably turns a lot of people off. Many people have too much of their identity wrapped up in the diet they identify with, whether it is vegan, vegetarian, low-carb, ketogenic, Paleo, or any of the other popular diet trends, so much so that it almost becomes a religious designation for some. If we are going to have a pragmatic and objective discussion about diet, I do not think it should be so dogmatic. We don't need a label. What we need is good, clean, wholesome food.

Second, is there any benefit to excluding animal products from the diet altogether? The honest answer is, we don't know. It is clear that methionine—which is found in high amounts in animal protein—is a significant growth factor for cancer. So if you have cancer, it seems prudent to limit high methionine foods, or even perhaps exclude them altogether. But will a piece of fish or grass-fed beef once a week alter a cancer patient's outcome? I don't believe so. However, that conversation with my patients can quickly devolve into, "How much can I have? How often?" I do not have a good answer for that, and I do not believe we can tease that answer out of the medical literature. Research studies show possible anti-cancer benefits from various dietary approaches, but no conclusive data. There are several reasons for this, including the fact that much of the nutrition research conducted is funded by special-interest groups and/or heavily biased to achieve a desired outcome.

If we are honest, there is still so much we do not know about diet and nutrition. We must balance that with pragmatic dietary advice that we *can* confidently offer. Thus, my recommendation is to always be plant-focused. However, different people tolerate changes to their diet in a variety of ways; therefore, I always encourage my patients to do their best and not get too stressed out if they "mess up" with their diet.

Preparing Your Own Food

Today, it has never been easier to delegate the responsibility of your food preparation and procurement. From take-out, to online delivery apps, to meal preparation programs, never has our access to food been easier, nor has what we eat been less our own responsibility than it is today. Whether that food is healthy or not, however, is not as clear. Even when you get "healthy" food from a restaurant, do you really know what is in it? For many people, their diet is exclusively food prepared by someone else. In these cases, it seems impossible to know what you are actually getting.

Relearning how to eat necessitates taking responsibility for what winds up on our plates. Largely, this means shopping for your own food and preparing it yourself. I recommend mostly shopping along the perimeter of the grocery store. The foods in these locations of the store tend to be less processed and generally healthier.

Shifting to this way of thinking about our food can be difficult for many people. Thankfully, there are many online tools available that may be beneficial. These include online databases of healthy recipes, meal plans, calorie trackers, and many more.

References

(1) Garber, J. E., and K. Offit. "Hereditary Cancer Predisposition Syndromes." *Journal of Clinical Oncology: Official Journal of the American Society of Clinical Oncology*. US National Library of Medicine, 10 Jan. 2005. Web. 02 July 2017.

(2) Song, Mingyang, and Edward Giovannucci. "Preventable Incidence and Mortality of Carcinoma Associated with Lifestyle Factors Among White Adults in the United States." *JAMA Oncology* 2.9 (2016): 1154. Web.

(3) Collective, The Tincture. "Nutrition and Cancer: Where Do We Go from Here? – Tincture." *Tincture*, 4 Mar. 2016, tincture.io/nutrition-and-cancer-where-do-we-go-from-here-7f93632e0464. Accessed 21 Aug. 2017.

(4) Doerr, Anne. "Using Only Alternative Medicine for Cancer Linked to Lower Survival Rate." *YaleNews*, 10 Aug. 2017, news.yale.edu/2017/08/10/using-only-alternative-medicine-cancer-linked-lower-survival-rate. Accessed 21 Aug. 2017.

CHAPTER 6

Your Nutritional Foundation

I encourage my patients to focus on including certain foods in their diet. By focusing on certain foods instead of worrying solely about what foods you should be excluding, it is much easier to cultivate a healthy, sensible approach to eating that is beneficial against cancer. Below are the foods I encourage my patients to focus on eating.

Vegetables

The bulk of the diet should be comprised of vegetables, especially green, leafy, and cruciferous vegetables such as spinach, kale, broccoli, brussels sprouts, cauliflower, and cabbage. (1) Cruciferous vegetables are rich in sulfuric compounds known as *glucosinolates*, which are known to have an anti-cancer effect. Other vegetables, such as squash, sweet potatoes, beets, carrots, and asparagus, are all great options as well. Generally speaking, vegetables are exceedingly rich in vitamins, minerals, phytonutrients, and fiber.

The possibilities here are endless. The advice to "eat the rainbow" of various colors of vegetables is spot on, as this adds variety to the diet and provides a wide spectrum of nutrients.

Here are some great vegetables to include in your diet: asparagus, beets, bell peppers, broccoli, brussels sprouts, cabbage, carrots, cauliflower, celery, collard greens, corn, cucumbers, eggplant, green beans, kale, leeks, mushrooms, mustard greens, okra, onions, parsley, peas, pumpkin, romaine lettuce, spinach, squash, sweet potatoes, swiss chard, turnip greens, watercress, white potatoes, and zucchini.

Fruits

Similar to vegetables, you will find an abundance of nutrition in fruits of all varieties. Some people express concern about fruits because of the high levels of naturally-occurring fructose—the form of sugar most abundant in fruits. Fructose can spike your insulin levels, but the presence of fiber also inherent in fruit works to mitigate this spike, making fruit safer to consume than foods that simply contain lots of added sugar or simple carbohydrates. In addition, the abundance of vitamins, minerals, antioxidants, and other beneficial compounds are all things we want to include regularly in our diet.

As is the case with vegetables, there are many wonderful fruits that can be helpful additions to the diet. These include apples, apricots, avocados, bananas, blackberries, blueberries, cantaloupe, coconuts, cranberries, dates, figs, grapefruit, grapes, honeydew melon, kiwi, lemons, limes, mangoes, nectarines, olives, oranges, papayas, peaches, pears, pineapples, plantains, plums, raisins, raspberries, strawberries, tangerines, tomatoes, and watermelon.

Fruits such as berries, apples, tomatoes, and avocados are packed with nutrition and also provide more fiber, resulting in a less substantial effect on blood sugar levels. Conversely, fruits such as melons, bananas, and pineapples should be enjoyed with slightly more moderation since they cause a sharper rise in blood sugar. This isn't to say that these fruits are forbidden, but simply that they should probably be consumed less often than some of the other fruits.

It is clear that a diet high in fruits and vegetables is essential for health as well as cancer prevention. A long-term study known as the Women's Health Initiative followed 50,000 women over a nearly 20-year period and found that women who increased their intake of fruits, vegetables, and whole grains while decreasing their intake of meats and cheeses saw a reduced risk of death following breast cancer. These women also slowed their progression of diabetes and prevented coronary heart disease, as compared to women who ate a diet higher in animal products and lower in plants. (2)

Raw vs. Cooked Foods

This is a good time to talk about the benefits of raw versus cooked food. We know that eating raw fruits and vegetables is good for us, but is it necessary to consume an *exclusively* raw diet? There is no doubt that such diets are incredibly nutritious, but I do not believe that an all-raw diet is necessary or practical.

However, there are some key foods that are ideally consumed raw. These include broccoli, cabbage, garlic, and onions.

One study measured levels of glucosinolates and sulforaphane in broccoli in humans after ingestion of raw and steamed broccoli. The levels of these anti-cancer constituents were found to be higher in those who ate raw broccoli than those who consumed steamed broccoli. (3) Another study that examined broccoli found that consumption of raw broccoli resulted in faster absorption and higher bioavailability of sulforaphane compared to cooked broccoli. (4)

Cabbage is important because it contains the enzyme *myrosinase*, which has documented anti-cancer activity. Research has shown that levels of myrosinase are higher in raw cabbage than in cooked cabbage. As little as two minutes of microwaving and seven minutes of steaming resulted in a complete loss of myrosinase activity. (5)

Garlic contains allyl sulfur compounds which have been shown to have anti-cancer properties. When garlic is cooked, these sulfur compounds are destroyed. Thus, eating garlic raw is ideal for preserving this key enzyme known as *alliinase*. However, one study found that crushed garlic allowed to sit at room temperature for ten minutes before microwaving for no more than 60 seconds prevented the total loss of anti-cancer activity. The levels of alliinase in the microwaved garlic were still much less than those found in raw garlic. (6)

Like garlic, onions are in the *Allium* family and contain potent anti-cancer elements. (7) Onions have been shown to inhibit the ability of platelets—the sticky component in the blood which helps a blood clot to form—from clumping together. This is important since platelet clumping, or *aggregation*, is a main step in the process of various ailments, including cancer, heart disease, and stroke. Studies have shown that when onions are steamed for three to six minutes, their anti-platelet activity is destroyed. Some other beneficial effects of onions remained when steaming occurred, but raw seems to be best. (8)

Interestingly, studies have shown that some foods are better for us when they are cooked. For example, *lycopene*, an important nutrient found in tomatoes, becomes more bioavailable when tomatoes are cooked. (9) Other foods, such as asparagus, carrots, mushrooms, and spinach, are also better for us when they are cooked. When asparagus is heated, its thick cell wall is broken down, allowing its constituent vitamins and minerals to be better absorbed by the body. (10) Carrots contain *beta carotene*, a known antioxidant and cancer fighter. It turns out that cooked carrots contain more beta carotene than raw carrots. (11) Mushrooms contain a potential carcinogen known as *agaritine*. Cooking mushrooms not only helps degrade agaritine but also releases an antioxidant known as *ergothioneine*. (12)

Spinach also seems to be best consumed after being cooked. One study found that steamed spinach retains more folate content while also reducing oxalic acid levels significantly. (13) *Oxalic acid*—also known as *oxalate*—inhibits absorption of essential nutrients and contributes to the majority of kidney stones. Thus, reducing oxalic acid is a good thing.

The point here is not to become bogged down with rules and regulations regarding which foods to eat raw and which foods to eat cooked. This is not a dos and don'ts list, especially since most foods that are better to eat raw are still nutritious when cooked, and vice versa. This section is merely included to illustrate the fact that a mix of raw and cooked food in the diet is ideal.

Finally, if you are eating animal protein, it is important to eat these foods only when they are cooked in order to mitigate the risk of food-borne illness.

Beans

Legumes such as black beans, pinto beans, chickpeas, lentils, and others are high in protein, complex carbohydrates, and a myriad of other nutrients. Populations that consume lots of beans have been observed to have a lower risk of developing cancer. (14) Beans have the benefit of being affordable and easy to store for long periods of time, particularly in raw/dry or canned form.

You might be wondering if consuming canned food is bad for you, since there has been much debate about this in recent years. Research dating back nearly 75 years has shown that foods retain their nutrient levels after the canning process. (15) However, some researchers have raised concerns about the levels of bisphenol-A (BPA) in canned foods, especially since BPA has been linked to various health problems. One study that evaluated many different canned foods identified BPA in roughly 90% of them. (16) A safe level of BPA has not been established, but my recommendation is to eat canned food sparingly without feeling the need to avoid it completely. Occasionally eating canned food is not likely to be harmful, but it probably isn't something you want to be consuming on a daily basis.

Grains

The grains that we should focus on are whole, minimally processed grains such as oats, quinoa, buckwheat, and amaranth. Ancient and sprouted grains are okay for those who tolerate gluten.

Similar to fruit, the glycemic spike of whole grains is mitigated by the fiber content. Often, people consume grains in the form of white flour. White flour contains only the starchy component of grains, but the bran (which is the fiber and nutrient-rich component of grain) has been removed. Without the inherent fiber, we see the insulin spikes that are associated with foods like pasta and bread. Although white flour tastes great, it doesn't offer much in the way of nutritional value.

Grains, as well as vegetables, fruits, beans, and lentils, are naturally higher in carbohydrates. You might be wondering if dietary carbohydrates are a problem. You have probably heard that "cancer loves sugar" and wondered if you should be eating a low-carbohydrate diet to treat or prevent cancer. Subsequently, there has been a lot of press recently about the ketogenic diet, which is a very-low-carbohydrate diet. Most ketogenic diet prescriptions for cancer treatment are not only very low in carbohydrates but also very low in protein as well, to the tune of about 95% of calories coming from fat and the remaining 5% coming from very small amounts of protein and carbohydrates. In addition to being a very difficult diet to follow, it also has several key drawbacks.

The reality is that although cancer can use sugar (carbohydrates) for energy, it can also use proteins, fats, and even ketones for energy. After all, cancer cells are mutated normal cells, so they are highly adaptable and can use various macronutrients for energy. You can't "starve" cancer by limiting one macronutrient such as carbohydrates; cancer can—and will—adapt to using other readily available sources of energy.

Rather than viewing nutrition as a way to starve cancer, view it instead as a way to support an optimal anti-cancer environment in the body.

Nuts, Seeds, and Healthy Oils

Foods like nuts, seeds, and healthy varieties of oils are all good options for a cancer-fighting diet. Nuts and seeds are rich in fiber and healthy fats and can be a good source of protein. These foods are high in calories, which can be beneficial for cancer patients struggling with unwanted weight loss. While they are calorically dense, they are not nutritionally void.

Fat has been a much-maligned macronutrient in previous years, but there is plenty of evidence that consuming healthy fats is beneficial for health; these are critical if we want to experience our best health. Oils such as coconut oil, flax oil, and extra-virgin olive oil contain cancer-fighting nutrients. Avocados (and avocado oil) are a great source of monounsaturated fats.

Grass-fed butter also contains beneficial nutrients and can be a good option as well. More specifically, grass-fed butter contains conjugated linoleic acid (CLA), a fat naturally found primarily in meat and dairy from ruminant animals such as cows, goats, bison, sheep, and elk. CLA is naturally anti-inflammatory, but it has also been shown to block the development and spread of cancer. (17) One study found that women who ate significant amounts of CLA in their diets had a 60 percent reduction in their risk of developing breast cancer. (18)

Eating meat and dairy from grass-fed animals, as opposed to the more common grain-fed sources today, is critically important. Virtually all of the beef and dairy produced before 1950 was from grass-fed animals. In the 1950s, the feedlot industry was born, where animals were fed grains to speed up the growth and development of these animals. This resulted in a more profitable meat and dairy industry for commercial farmers, but unfortunately, it reduced the nutritional content of the final product. In fact, research has shown that grass-fed animals have three to five times more CLA than animals fed grain. (19)

You have probably wondered at some point if eating fat is bad for you, especially since dietary fat has been vilified for decades. One study suggested that fat intake in young women might be linked to an increased risk of breast cancer. However, the increased risk seen in this study was attributed specifically to animal fat and not vegetable fat. (20) Another study suggested a link between high consumption of beef, pork, and lamb and an increased risk of colon cancer. (21) The conclusion from these studies was that there was something specific in the animal fat which caused the increased risk of cancer. I believe it was the fat from grain-fed, hormone-supplemented animals these test subjects were almost certainly consuming which led to the increased cancer risk. In other words, animal fat in its natural, grass-fed, organic form isn't the problem. The problem is the way modern farming and manufacturing has altered these otherwise nutritious foods.

Aside from the aforementioned study that suggested a link between fat consumption and an increased cancer risk, we have many studies showing just the opposite. A large study that followed over 88,000 women for a period of nearly 15 years found no evidence that a lower intake of dietary fat resulted in a decreased risk of breast cancer. (22) Another large study examined the effect of a low-fat diet on the risk of colorectal cancer and found that women who ate a low-fat diet had no decreased risk of colorectal compared to those who did not. (23)

My recommendation is to neither be afraid of dietary fat nor go out of your way to eat a lot of it. The research does not point to a need to eat a low-fat diet or a high-fat diet. Focus on naturally occurring fats in their whole, unprocessed, or minimally processed form, and you will be fine. Just don't eat them at the exclusion of healthy, organic plants such as vegetables, fruits, and grains.

Herbs and Spices

A wide variety of herbs and spices are known to promote health, and many of these have been shown to have anti-cancer benefits. These include herbs and spices such as thyme, cinnamon, cloves, turmeric, cumin, oregano, sage, parsley, rosemary, mint, lavender, garlic, dill, cilantro, chives, and basil. These are just a few, and there are many others! We should include these liberally in our food. (24, 25)

Most Americans are accustomed to eating a diet rich in fat, sugar, and salt; these are all flavors our bodies are engineered to crave. The presence of fat and sugar in food is a signal to our body that the food we are tasting is high in calories and, thus, high in energy. And while many people consume too much sodium, it is a very important nutrient for biochemical processes in our body. For our hunter-gatherer ancestors, the sense of taste was valuable for survival and drove them to seek out these types of flavors. This explains why these nutrients are so addictive; our body is designed to crave them. Unfortunately, this has negative implications for the way people eat today.

Instead of relying simply on salt, sugar, and high-fat foods for delicious flavor, herbs and spices can add complexity and flavor to our foods while conferring numerous health benefits. Particularly herbs and spices such as turmeric, oregano, garlic, black cumin, saffron, black pepper, and chili pepper have all been observed to have potent anti-cancer effects. (26) Although many of these are available as nutritional supplements in capsule form, I encourage everyone to use these spices in cooking as much as possible. After all, they were used medicinally in food long before they could be manufactured into a supplement.

Beverages

Proper hydration is essential for optimal functioning of the body's cells, tissues, and organs. Water should unequivocally be your beverage of choice. Drinking water on the go has become common in recent years as people have become more aware of the importance of hydration; bottled water has become a lucrative industry, and many people are now taking a thermos of water with them as they go about their day. But how much water should we really be drinking?

A group of researchers set out to determine an optimal amount of water consumption per day and arrived at approximately 3,000 milliliters (100 fluid ounces) per day for men and 2,200 milliliters (75 fluid ounces) per day for women. These researchers pointed out that water consumption beyond this point was not helpful, and could in fact be harmful for certain people. (27) Another guideline, which is perhaps slightly more accurate for each individual, is to aim for approximately half your body weight in fluid ounces every day. Therefore, if you weigh 200 pounds, you should try to drink 100 fluid ounces of water daily. This is not a hard-and-fast rule, but a general framework to ensure that you are staying hydrated. Some people will need more, and others will need less, depending on person-to-person variations in physiology, climate, and activity level.

Drinking water by itself is great, but if you simply don't like plain water, don't despair. You can liven up your plain water by squeezing a lemon or lime into it. Exercise caution when relying on adding flavored powders to your water, as many contain artificial sweeteners such as sucralose and aspartame.

I recommend caution when consuming bottled water, whether it be still water or carbonated water. A recent study found that many drinking water brands on the market contain elevated levels of a group of manmade chemicals known as *polyfluoroalkyl substances* (PFAS). These chemicals are ubiquitous in the environment today as a result of their widespread use in industry since the 1950s, including nonstick cookware, stain-repellent carpets, and cleaning products. Because of this, they make their way into our water supply. Today, drinking water is one of the most common routes of exposure to PFAS. This is important because exposure to high levels of PFAS has been linked to potential health issues, including cancer, heart disease, liver dysfunction, and pregnancy complications.

In a recent study, multiple samples of 47 bottled water brands (35 non-carbonated and 12 carbonated) found that many had PFAS levels above the recommended amounts. (28) While occasional exposure to PFAS is unlikely to be harmful, routine consumption of bottled water could lead to health problems. For this reason, I recommend exercising caution.

What about tap water? Although the water from your tap has certainly been treated to some degree to remove obvious contaminants and pollutants, this is no guarantee that it is as clean as you might think. The Environmental Working Group tested water samples from throughout the United States and found more than 250 contaminants! (29) Simply put, the current safety standards for tap water are not based on the most updated scientific recommendations for health and safety.

The ideal solution is to have a really good water filtration system at home. A whole-house water filtration system that filters out multiple types of contaminants, including heavy metals, chlorine, and pesticides is ideal, as it not only purifies the water you drink but also the water you use to wash your hands and bathe. Filtering your water properly at home provides the assurance that the majority of the water you consume is good for you rather than being harmful in any capacity.

Tea is another excellent beverage that can be enjoyed. Green tea is especially noteworthy, as it contains a substance called *epigallocatechin-3-gallate*, also known as *EGCG*. Green tea is thought to play a role in cancer prevention (30) and in suppressing tumor cell growth. (31) *Essiac tea*, which contains slippery elm, burdock root, sheep sorrel, and Indian rhubarb, is known as an anti-cancer tea. (32)

Coffee is another beverage I highly recommend. Although it has been a polarizing beverage through the years, we now have some compelling studies suggesting a strong anti-cancer benefit from coffee. Most of the research has been done on the natural, caffeinated version, which is what I recommend for those who can tolerate caffeine. Decaffeinated coffee seems to have similar anti-cancer benefits, but the decaffeinating process can introduce harsh chemicals, so caution is warranted. Choosing organic coffee, whether caffeinated or decaffeinated, is very important.

One study found that coffee reduces the risk of brain cancer by 40%. (33) Another found that at least two cups of coffee per day reduced colon cancer risk. (34) Yet another found that at least three cups of coffee daily prevented or delayed the onset of certain cancers in women, including breast, colon, lung, and ovarian cancers. (35)

Consuming coffee "black," without any additives such as cream, half and half, or sugar, is best. However, if you must sweeten your coffee, opt for stevia.

As for how much coffee to consume, the sweet spot based on research seems to be between two and four cups per day. Please remember that caffeine is a drug, so treat it with respect. If you're relying on coffee to wake up in the morning or to make it through the day, I suggest taking a closer look at your sleep habits and stress levels.

Seven Superfoods

Superfoods are foods with purportedly numerous health benefits, although the term is a bit nebulous. In other words, there is no general consensus on what actually constitutes a *superfood*. However, for our purposes, I have identified seven foods with noteworthy anti-cancer properties. These are foods we should regularly include in our diets to glean the anti-cancer benefits therein.

1. Garlic

Garlic is among the most potent of cancer-fighting foods we have available. Studies show that garlic not only prevents cancer but also kills multiple different types of cancer cells. In a study of over 30 vegetable extracts and their ability to inhibit the growth of multiple cancers, garlic was successful in halting every kind of cancer. (36) Other foods in the same family as garlic with similar anti-cancer benefits are green onions, yellow onions, and leeks.

2. Broccoli

Broccoli contains sulforaphane and indole-3-carbinol, both of which are potent cancer-fighting substances. Sulforaphane has been rigorously studied and is particularly important because it targets cancer stem cells (CSCs). (37) Cancer stem cells are a small but important subpopulation of cancer cells within tumors, noteworthy because they have the ability for self-renewal, differentiation, and tumorigenicity. (38)

Broccoli is a cruciferous vegetable belonging to the same family as brussels sprouts, cauliflower, kale, and red cabbage. All of these are beneficial foods when it comes to preventing cancer, but none are quite as rich in sulforaphane as broccoli. You can also enjoy broccoli sprouts.

3. Carrots
Carrots are rich in carotenoids, including alpha- and beta-carotene, as well as bioflavonoids. Studies indicate that carrots reduce inflammation, improve immune system function, and kill cancer cells. (39)

4. Beets
The characteristic red color associated with beets is derived from betalain, which has been shown to starve tumors and hinder cell division. Beets have been found in studies to exhibit direct cancer-killing behaviors. (40)

5. Ginger
Ginger is beneficial against cancer in a variety of ways. It has been shown to kill various types of cancer cells in lab studies. It has been shown to modulate the expression of genes, scavenge for free radicals, and induce apoptosis (programmed cell death) of cancer cells. (41) As an added benefit, ginger is an excellent natural treatment for nausea.

6. Tomatoes
The nutrient responsible for tomatoes' bright red color, lycopene, is a carotenoid that is well-documented for its ability to prevent cancer. (42) Tomatoes can be enjoyed raw or in homemade sauce and salsa. As mentioned earlier, there is evidence that cooking tomatoes makes lycopene more bioavailable. (43)

7. Cranberries

In a study designed to investigate the ability of various fruits to reduce oxidative damage and slow the proliferation of cancer, cranberries were the clear winner in both categories. (44) Cranberries are rich in ellagic acid, anthocyanidins, proanthocyanidins, and polyphenols, all of which are known to inhibit the growth of tumors.

Along with cranberries, I recommend including blueberries, strawberries, raspberries, and blackberries in the diet. All these berries come with many of the same anti-cancer benefits cranberries possess.

References

(1) Higdon J., et al. "Cruciferous Vegetables and Human Cancer Risk: Epidemiologic Evidence and Mechanistic Basis." *Pharmacological Research*, vol. 55, no. 3, 2007, pp. 224–236., doi:10.1016/j.phrs.2007.01.009.

(2) Prentice R.L., Aragaki A.K., Howard B.V., et al. "Low-Fat Dietary Pattern among Postmenopausal Women Influences Long-Term Cancer, Cardiovascular Disease, and Diabetes Outcomes." *J Nutr* 2019; 149(9): 1565–74. doi: 10.1093/jn/nxz107.

(3) Conaway C.C., Getahun S.M., Liebes L.L., et al. "Disposition of Glucosinolates and Sulforaphane in Humans after Ingestion of Steamed and Fresh Broccoli." *Nutr Cancer* 2000; 38(2): 168-78. doi: 10.1207/S15327914NC382_5.

(4) Vermeulen M., Klopping-Ketelaars I.W., van den Berg R., and Vaes W.H. "Bioavailability and Kinetics of Sulforaphane in Humans after Consumption of Cooked Versus Raw Broccoli." *J Agric Food Chem* 2008; 56(22): 10505-9. doi: 10.1021/jf801989e.

(5) Rungapamestry V., Duncan A.J., Fuller Z., and Ratcliffe B. "Changes in Glucosinolate Concentrations, Myrosinase Activity, and Production of Metabolites of Glucosinolates in Cabbage (Brassica Oleracea Var. Capitata) Cooked for Different Durations." *J Agric Food Chem* 2006; 54(20): 7628-34. doi: 10.1021/jf0607314.

(6) Song K., Milner J.A. "The Influence of Heating on the Anticancer Properties of Garlic." *J Nutr* 2001; 131(3s): 1054S-7S. doi: 10.1093/jn/131.3.1054S.

(7) Nicastro H.L., Ross S.A., Milner J.A. "Garlic and Onions: Their Cancer Prevention Properties." *Cancer Prev Res (Phila)* 2015; 8(3): 181-9. doi: 10.1158/1940-6207.CAPR-14-0172.

(8) Hansen E.A., Folts J.D., Goldman I.L. "Steam-Cooking Rapidly Destroys and Reverses Onion-Induced Antiplatelet Activity." *Nutr J* 2012; 11: 76. doi: 10.1186/1475-2891-11-76.

(9) Dewanto V., Wu X., Adom K.K., Liu R.H. "Thermal Processing Enhances the Nutritional Value of Tomatoes by Increasing Total Antioxidant Activity." *J Agric Food Chem* 2002; 50(10): 3010-4. doi: 10.1021/jf0115589.

(10) Miglio C., Chiavaro E., Visconti A., et al. "Effects of Different Cooking Methods on Nutritional and Physicochemical Characteristics of Selected Vegetables." *J Agric Food Chem* 2008; 56(1): 139-47. doi: 10.1021/jf072304b.

(11) Talcott S.T., Howard L.R., Brenes C.H. "Antioxidant Changes and Sensory Properties of Carrot Puree Processed with and without Periderm Tissue." *J Agric Food Chem* 2000; 48(4): 1351-21. doi: 10.1021/jf9910178.

(12) Schulzová V., Hajslová J., Peroutka R., et al. "Influence of Storage and Household Processing on the Agaritine Content of the Cultivated Agaricus Mushroom." *Food Addit Contam* 2002; 19(9): 853-62. doi: 10.1080/02652030210156340) Martin K.R. "The Bioactive Agent Ergothioneine, a Key Component of Dietary Mushrooms, Inhibits Monocyte Binding to Endothelial Cells Characteristic of Early Cardiovascular Disease." *J Med Food* 2010; 13(6): 1340-6. doi: 10.1089/jmf.2009.0194.

(13) Chai W., Liebman M. "Effect of Different Cooking Methods on Vegetable Oxalate Content." *J Agric Food Chem* 2005; 53(8): 3027-30. doi: 10.1021/jf048128d.

(14) Campos-Vega, Rocio, et al. "Common Beans and Their Non-Digestible Fraction: Cancer Inhibitory Activity—An Overview." *Foods*, vol. 2, no. 3, 2013, pp. 374–392., doi:10.3390/foods2030374.

(15) Cameron E.J., Pilcher R.W., Clifcorn L.E. "Nutrient Retention During Canned Food Production." *Am J Public Health Nations Health* 1949; 39(6): 756-63. doi:10.2105/ajph.39.6.756.

(16) Noonan G.O., Ackerman L.K., Begley T.H. "Concentration of Bisphenol A in Highly Consumed Canned Foods on the US Market." *J Agric Food Chem* 2011; 59(13): 7178-85. doi: 10.1021/jf201076f.

(17) Ip C., Scimeca J.A., Thompson H.J. "Conjugated Linoleic Acid. A Powerful Anticarcinogen from Animal Fat Sources." *Cancer* 1994; 74(3 Suppl): 1050-4. doi: 10.1002/1097-0142 (19940801) 74:3+<1050::aid-cncr2820741512>3.0.co;2-i.

(18) Aro A., Männistö S., Salminen I., et al. "Inverse Association Between Dietary and Serum Conjugated Linoleic Acid and Risk of Breast Cancer in Postmenopausal Women." *Nutr Cancer* 2000; 38(2): 151-7. doi: 10.1207/S15327914NC382_2.

(19) Dhiman T.R., Anand G.R., Satter L.D., et al. "Conjugated Linoleic Acid Content of Milk from Cows Fed Different Diets." *J Dairy Sci* 1999; 82(10): 2146-56. doi: 10.3168/jds.S0022-0302(99)75458-5.

(20) Cho E., Spiegelman D., Hunter D.J., Chen W.Y., Stampfer M.J., Colditz G.A., Willett W.C. "Premenopausal Fat Intake and Risk of Breast Cancer." *J Natl Cancer Inst* 2003; 95(14): 1079-85. doi: 10.1093/jnci/95.14.1079.

(21) Clinton S.K., Giovannucci E.L., Hursting S.D. "The World Cancer Research Fund/American Institute for Cancer Research Third Expert Report on Diet, Nutrition, Physical Activity, and Cancer: Impact and Future Directions." *J Nutr* 2020; 150(4): 663-71. doi: 10.1093/jn/nxz268.

(22) "Holmes M.D., Hunter D.J., Colditz G.A., et al. Association of Dietary Intake of Fat and Fatty Acids with Risk of Breast Cancer." *JAMA* 1999; 281(10): 914-20. doi: 10.1001/jama.281.10.914.

(23) Beresford S.A., Johnson K.C., Ritenbaugh C., et al. "Low-Fat Dietary Pattern and Risk of Colorectal Cancer: The Women's Health Initiative Randomized Controlled Dietary Mod-

ification Trial." *JAMA* 2006; 295(6): 643-54. doi: 10.1001/jama.295.6.643.

(24) Kaefer, Christine M., and John A. Milner. "The Role of Herbs and Spices in Cancer Prevention." *The Journal of Nutritional Biochemistry*, vol. 19, no. 6, 2008, pp. 347–361., doi:10.1016/j.jnutbio.2007.11.003.

(25) Kaefer, Christine M., and John A. Milner. "Chapter 17 Herbs and Spices in Cancer Prevention and Treatment." *Herbal Medicine: Biomolecular and Clinical Aspects.*, 2nd ed., CRC Press/Taylor & Francis, 2011.

(26) Zheng J., Zhou Y., Li Y., et al. "Spices for Prevention and Treatment of Cancers." *Nutrients* 2016; 8(8): 495. doi:10.3390/nu8080495.

(27) Meinders A.J., Meinders A.E. "How Much Water Do We Really Need to Drink?" *Ned Tijdschr Geneeskd* 2010; 154: A1757. Dutch.

(28) Felton A. "What's Really in Your Bottled Water?" https://www.consumerreports.org/bottled-water/whats-really-in-your-bottled-water. Accessed February 21, 2021.

(29) "Meets All Government Standards: EWG's Tap Water Database Details Unsafe Contamination in Communities Nationwide." https://www.ewg.org/release/meets-all-government-standards-ewg-s-2019-tap-water-database-details-unsafe-contamination. Accessed February 21, 2021.

(30) Liu J., Xing J., and Fei Y. "Green Tea (*Camellia sinensis*) and Cancer Prevention: A Systematic Review Of Randomized Trials And Epidemiological Studies." *Chin Med* 2008; 3: 12.

(31) Zhao T., Sun Q., del Rincon S.V., ,et al. "Gallotannin imposes S Phase Arrest in Breast Cancer Cells and Suppresses the Growth of Triple Negative Tumors in Vivo." *PLoS One* 2014; 9(3): e92853.

(32) Leonard S.S., Keil D., Mehlman T., et al. "Essiac Tea: Scavenging of Reactive Oxygen Species and Effects on DNA Damage." *J Ethnopharmacol* 2006; 103(2): 288-96. doi: 10.1016/j.jep.2005.09.013.

(33) Holick C.N., Smith S.G., Giovannucci E., et al. "Coffee, Tea, Caffeine Intake, and Risk of Adult Glioma in Three Prospective Cohort Studies." *Cancer Epidemiol Biomarkers* Prev 2010; 19(1): 39-47.

(34) Oba S., Shimizu N.., Nagata C, et al. "The Relationship Between the Consumption of Meat, Fat, and Coffee and the Risk of Colon Cancer: A Prospective Study in Japan." *Cancer Letters* 2006; 244 (2): 260-67.

(35) Lukic M., Licaj I., Lund E., et al. "Coffee Consumption and the Risk of Cancer in the Norwegian Women and Cancer (NOWAC) Study." *Eur J Epidemiol* 2016; 31(9): 905-16.

(36) Boivin D., Lamy S., Lord-Dufour S., et al. "Antiproliferative and Antioxidant Activities of Common Vegetables: A Comparative Study." *Food Chemistry* 2009; 112: 374-380.

(37) Li Y., Zhang T. "Targeting Cancer Stem Cells with Sulforaphane, a Dietary Component from Broccoli and Broccoli Sprouts." *Future Oncol* 2013; 9(8): 1097-1103.

(38) Yu Z., Pestell T.G., Lisanti M.P., Pestell R.G. "Cancer Stem Cells." *Int J Biochem Cell Biol* 2012; 44(12): 2144-51. doi:10.1016/j.biocel.2012.08.022.

(39) da Silva Dias J. "Nutritional and Health Benefits of Carrots and Their Seed Extracts." *Food and Nutr Sci* 2014; 5: 2147-56.

(40) Kapadia G.J., Azuine M.A., Rao G.S., et al. "Cytotoxic Effect of the Red Beetroot (*Beta vulgaris L.*) Extract Compared to Doxorubicin (Adriamycin) in the Human Prostate (PC-3) and Breast (MCF-7) Cancer Cell Lines." *Anticancer Agents Med Chem* 2011; 11(3): 280-4.

(41) Baliga M.S., Haniadka R., Pereira M.M., et al. "Update on the Chemopreventative Effects of Ginger and Its Phytochemicals." *Crit Rev Fod Sci Nutr* 2011; 51(6): 499-523.

(42) Dahan K., Fennal M., Kumar N.B. "Lycopene in the Prevention of Prostate Cancer. *J Soc Integr Oncol* 2008; 6(1): 29-36.

(43) Cornell University. "Cooking Tomatoes Boosts Disease-Fighting Power." ScienceDaily. 23 April 2002. <www.sciencedaily.com/releases/2002/04/020422073341.htm>.

(44) Sun J., Chu Y.F., Wu X., and Liu R.H. "Antioxidant and Antiproliferative Activities of Common Fruits." *J Agric Food Chem* 2002; 50(25): 7449-54.

CHAPTER 7

What to Eat in Moderation

In the interest of cultivating a nutrition plan designed to fight cancer, some foods are shown to be neither inherently good nor inherently bad. These foods should be enjoyed in moderation. If you enjoy them, feel free to include them in your nutrition plan on a somewhat restricted basis. If you don't enjoy them, or if you have a hard time limiting the amounts of these foods, it is certainly fine to eliminate them entirely.

If you have an ethical or religious belief that prevents you from consuming a substance on this list, that's okay. None of these foods are essential for a healthy, anti-cancer lifestyle. With that said, some of these foods do provide benefits, so if you leave any of these out of your diet entirely, you might need to achieve these benefits in other ways.

Alcohol

Alcohol is considered by some to be a forbidden substance because we know that drinking too much might actually cause cancer. When alcohol breaks down in the body, a byproduct called *acetaldehyde* is formed. Acetaldehyde is known to damage DNA as well as proteins in the body. Too much alcohol also increases fat storage and estrogen, an important factor in many different types of cancer.

What does the research tell us? A landmark study followed roughly 100,000 adults aged 55–74 for an average of nine years to assess a relationship between alcohol intake and cancer development. Researchers found that those who never consumed alcohol were at the lowest risk of developing cancer, compared to those who were light-moderate or heavy drinkers. Not surprisingly, the heavy drinkers were at the highest risk of developing cancer. The same linear relationship existed between the amount of alcohol consumption and cancer death. (1)

It is important to note that the study above showed an association between alcohol and cancer death and did not prove cause and effect. In other words, we are dealing with correlation and not necessarily causation.

Another study found that low to moderate alcohol intake, defined as one glass of wine per day for women and two glasses of wine per day for men, was associated with a small but insignificant increase in cancer overall. (2)

Alcohol doesn't provide any tangible health benefits, and the research suggests that moderate to heavy intake of alcohol increases the risk of multiple health problems, including cancer. So let's be clear: You don't need alcohol, and consuming it does constitute some level of risk.

With that said, light alcohol consumption has not been shown to have any appreciable impact on cancer development. If you choose to consume alcohol, I recommend restricting it to one drink per day at the most. A drink is defined as 5 fluid ounces of wine, 12 fluid ounces of beer, and 1.5 fluid ounces of 80-proof liquor.

Unfortunately, the research into alcohol's impact on patients already diagnosed with cancer is lacking. Because alcohol does not provide any anti-cancer benefit, I think it makes sense to follow the guidelines above, or perhaps restrict consumption further. If you are currently undergoing cancer treatment, please consult your physician regarding alcohol consumption, as alcohol can interact with certain medicines you may be taking.

Dairy

Dairy products such as milk, cheese, butter, cream, and yogurt are commonplace in many diets around the world. A significant amount of research has been performed to examine a possible relationship between dairy and cancer. It is important to note that this research, like most nutrition research, is typically observational in nature. Observational studies *observe* people's eating habits and follow those people over time to see if they develop a specific health outcome. These studies tell us if a person is more or less likely to get a disease, but they cannot *prove* that a food caused a disease. Thus, these studies are limited in terms of drawing conclusions, but they do provide clues.

A recent study found that intake of as little as 1/4 cup of dairy milk per day was associated with an increased risk of breast cancer. Drinking more, up to 1 cup of dairy milk per day, increased the risk of breast cancer further. (3) One of the study authors stated that the sex hormone content of dairy milk could be the reason for the increased breast cancer risk seen.

Another study found that women with breast cancer who consumed high-fat dairy had a greater risk of death compared to those who consumed low-fat dairy. (4) The evidence regarding dairy intake and breast cancer, however, is not clear-cut. A review of 52 studies found no association between dairy consumption and the risk of breast cancer. (5)

Another study evaluated the impact of dairy consumption on prostate cancer risk. The study found a relationship between high intakes of dairy products, including milk and cheese, and a possibly increased risk of prostate cancer. (6)

To further complicate matters, a recent meta-analysis found that high dairy consumption was associated with a lower risk of developing colorectal cancer as well as a lower risk of dying from colorectal cancer. This study combined the results of 31 studies and included nearly 25,000 patients. In other words, it was a strong and well-powered study.

One group of researchers recognized the need for high-quality research on the topic of dairy consumption and cancer. They identified over 8,000 individual research papers on the topic of dairy and cancer, published between 1991 and 2017. As expected, the quality of these studies varied widely. After excluding the studies which did not meet their criteria for quality, they found that 71% showed no evidence of a statistically significant association between dairy consumption and cancer development. In addition, 16% of studies showed an increased risk of cancer with dairy consumption, and 13% showed decreased risk of cancer with dairy consumption. (7)

As we can see, studies on dairy and cancer have largely been inconclusive, due to the fact that dairy products comprise a large food group. (8)

The scientific evidence does not point to dairy needing to be eliminated completely. However, I do feel that a case can be made to limit it. When you do consume dairy, it is best to consume organic, grass-fed dairy products raised without hormones. Part of the concern I have with conventional dairy products is the widespread use of recombinant bovine growth hormone (rBGH). Typically, cows are grown using hormones and antibiotics, which subsequently harms the cows and contaminates meat and dairy products. These products contain estrogenic compounds as well. Knowing that these contaminants seem to fuel the growth and development of multiple cancers, it seems prudent to be very selective when it comes to dairy consumption.

Goat dairy products are permissible as well. They can be a good option for those who have allergies or sensitivities to cow's milk. Please remember that goat milk still contains lactose, so if you are lactose intolerant, it is best to stick to plant-based milk products.

Meat and Seafood

As we have established, the foundation of an anti-cancer diet should be vegetables. We can round this out with fruits, nuts, grains, and seeds, along with some healthy dairy. Meat and seafood are a controversial topic, and one we must explore in our quest for the optimal anti-cancer diet.

First, we must establish some definitions. We will define *meat* as "flesh from warm-blooded animals such as cows, pigs, sheep, chickens, and birds." This category can be further subdivided into red meat, which includes beef, pork, lamb, veal, and mutton; and white meat, which includes chicken and turkey. We will define *seafood* as "flesh from cold-blooded animals such as salmon, tuna, mackerel, shrimp, and lobster."

Red Meat

The World Cancer Research Fund, in association with the American Institute for Cancer Research, has noted strong evidence for an association between red meat, as well as processed meat, and the development of colorectal cancer. Evidence for this recommendation includes a review of the existing literature on the topic, which found that consumption of red meat—and especially processed meat—was associated with an increased risk of cancers of the colon and rectum. (9)

Is red meat inherently bad? Or is our method of processing and/or preparing red meat the issue? I believe that red meat becomes potentially harmful when we distort it from what it was meant to be. For example, beef naturally comes from cows that are fed diets of grass, not grain, and which are allowed to reach their full size without the use of growth hormone and antibiotics. The beef industry of today relies heavily on these unnatural means to improve the quantity of meat produced. Research shows us that grass-fed beef has less fat overall than grain-fed beef, while having nearly five times the amount of beneficial omega-3 fats. (10) In addition, grass-fed beef contains more vitamins and antioxidants than its grain-fed counterpart. (11)

There is some confusion regarding labels and definitions, so let's discuss those. The United States Department of Agriculture (USDA) certifies organic beef. The USDA Certified Organic label tells us that the meat comes from cattle that have received 100% organic feed and forage. This means that they are not genetically modified (i.e., they are non-GMO). This also means that the cows were raised in living conditions that allowed them to graze in pastures. Finally, the organic certification also tells us that the cows were never administered antibiotics or hormones. Eat organic!

When you see a label that says that beef is grass fed, it means that the cows were fed grass at some point during their lives. Simply having "grass fed" on the label does *not* mean that the cows never received grain. Instead, look for "100% grass fed" on the label, which means that the cattle never received any grain.

An extra attribute to look for is *grass finished*. This means that the cows were not only fed grass throughout the growing period but also "finished" on a diet that was totally grass. If you just see "grass fed" on a label, but not "grass finished," it's safe to assume that those cows were grass fed for most of their lives but received grain for a period of time after that.

Meat that is conventionally raised comprises the vast majority of commercially produced beef. If the label doesn't say organic or grass fed, it's run-of-the-mill, conventionally produced. Conventionally raised cows are moved to a feedlot at approximately eight months of age, which is the time they are weaned from their mother's milk. These cows are fed grains, corn, and soy. This method produces fatter cows, resulting in more beef available for sale commercially.

One of the theories about why these conventionally raised cows are larger and fatter relates not only to what they are fed but also how they live. Most of these conventionally raised cows are kept in small spaces, which prevents their natural desire to graze. Some scientists speculate that this greatly increases the cows' stress levels, leading to increased cortisol. As we know, high cortisol leads to weight gain.

On the topic of meat preparation, we must acknowledge the fact that cooking meat at high temperatures introduces compounds such as heterocyclic amines (HCAs) and polycyclic aromatic hydrocarbons (PAHs). Studies have shown a relationship between the HCAs introduced when red meat is cooked well-done and the development of cancer. (12) Research into PAHs has shown a similar carcinogenic effect. (13)

Based on the many benefits of grass-fed beef and the fact that it is far less common than grain-fed beef in today's diets, I can't help but wonder if the negative health outcomes associated with red meat consumption are due to harmful contaminants introduced via modern farming and improper cooking practices.

Processed meat is a different story. When we refer to *processed meat*, we are referring to meat that has been treated in some way, such as meat that has been cured, salted, smoked, or chemically preserved in some way. Some examples of processed meat include hot dogs, bacon, sausage, salami, and pepperoni. Various organizations, including the International Agency for Research on Cancer (IARC), have declared processed meat a definite carcinogen. (14) Several types of cancer appear to be particularly associated with routine consumption of processed meats, including colorectal and stomach. The mechanism for this appears to occur as a result of cooking nitrates and nitrites in these meats at high temperatures. When exposed to heat, these components are converted into carcinogenic nitrosamines, which can damage healthy DNA, resulting in mutations that can lead to cancer.

White Meat

Poultry such as chicken and turkey are often considered to be healthier than red meat. This is historically due to the fact that white meat is lower in fat content. Interestingly, a meta-analysis that analyzed and compiled multiple studies found that there was an *inverse* association between poultry consumption and colorectal cancer. (15) An inverse relationship means that people who ate poultry were found to have a lower risk of cancer than those who did not. Other research has found a reduced risk of lung cancer in those who consume poultry. (16)

Some researchers have wondered if substituting chicken for red meat might have an impact on cancer development. One study found that people who kept their intake of meat consistent but replaced red meat with chicken saw a reduction in their risk of developing multiple cancers, including esophageal, lung, liver, and colorectal. The study authors found that simply increasing poultry intake without reducing the intake of red meat did not seem to reduce cancer risk. In other words, chicken itself didn't reduce cancer risk; eating less red meat did. (17)

Poultry isn't necessary, but eating it occasionally is probably fine.

Eggs

One study found that men who ate 2.5 or more eggs had an increased risk of advanced prostate cancer compared to men who ate less than 0.5 eggs per week. (18) This is thought to be due to the fact that eggs have a high choline content (even higher than other animal foods).

Another study found an increased risk of prostate, breast, and ovarian cancer in test subjects who consumed more than five eggs per week, compared to those who did not consume eggs at all. (19) This was thought to be due to the cholesterol content of eggs, since cholesterol is a required substrate for the production of hormones in the body (which can drive the growth of these cancers).

One study found an increased risk of cancers of the digestive tract in those who consume eggs. This was especially true with respect to colorectal cancer. (20)

You don't need eggs in your diet, but eating them occasionally is unlikely to be detrimental from a cancer perspective.

Seafood

When it comes to seafood, there are three main categories: fish, shellfish, and roe. Fish comprises many different options, with some examples including anchovies, bass, catfish, cod, eel, flounder, grouper, haddock, halibut, herring, mackerel, salmon, snapper, sole, swordfish, tilapia, trout, tuna, and whiting. Shellfish can be subdivided into crustaceans and mollusks. Crustaceans include crabs, crawfish, lobster, and shrimp. Mollusks include clams, mussels, octopuses, oysters, scallops, and squid. Roe includes caviar, lumpfish, and massage, among others.

Next, we must understand the difference between wild-caught fish and farmed fish. Wild-caught fish exist in the wild and eat their natural diets. In contrast, farmed fish (sometimes termed *aquaculture*) are produced under controlled conditions (tanks, oceans, lakes, or rivers) where they can be fed specific diets. It is estimated that approximately half of the seafood supply today comes from aquaculture. (21)

We must also consider pollution in the water in which the seafood lives. The Environmental Protection Agency (EPA) and the Food and Drug Administration (FDA) have issued advice about fish and shellfish, and they recommend women of childbearing age, women who are pregnant or breastfeeding, and young children to avoid several fish known to have higher mercury levels. These include king mackerel, shark, swordfish, tilefish, and tuna. (22)

In terms of seafood consumption and cancer risk, we have several enlightening studies to review. One study found that vegetarians who added fish to their diets further reduced their risk of colon cancer. More specifically, researchers found that eating a vegetarian diet resulted in a 22% reduced risk of colon cancer compared to non-vegetarians, but when these vegetarians added fish to their diets, the risk of colon cancer was reduced by 43%. (23) This combination seems to work well, since vegetarian diets often include many nutritious plants that provide high amounts of fiber, while the fish provide good dietary sources of omega-3 fats as well as vitamin D. This dietary approach also avoids red meat and pork, which as we know have been linked to an increased risk of colorectal cancer.

Another paper evaluated the bulk of the scientific literature on fish consumption and health outcomes and found that fish consumption reduced the risk of cancer as well as other health issues, including cardiovascular disease. (24) These researchers found that fish intake is generally safe, with the most benefits gained from consuming two to four servings of fish per week.

There have also been meta-analyses that concluded that fish consumption lowers the risk of lung cancer, (25) thyroid cancer, (26) and gastric cancer. (27)

Other studies have not found a cancer reduction benefit from fish consumption. These include studies evaluating fish consumption and prostate cancer, (28) breast cancer, (29) endometrial cancer, (30) and ovarian cancer. (31)

If you do choose to eat fish, there are several which seem to confer an especially high degree of health benefits. These include salmon, mackerel, sardines, trout, and herring.

Salmon has several health benefits, including omega-3 fats as well as many vitamins and minerals. It is important to choose wild-caught instead of farmed. Farmed salmon has been shown to have lower levels of omega-3s, vitamins, and minerals than wild-caught salmon. In addition, some research has shown that wild-caught salmon, especially from Alaska, has a significantly lower amount of contaminants such as dioxins, polychlorinated biphenyls, polybrominated biphenyl ethers, and pesticides compared to wild-caught salmon. (32) As is the case with beef, we should be consuming food from its natural state as much as possible. In this case, opt for wild-caught salmon over farmed salmon.

Mackerel contains a high amount of omega-3s. This is especially true of mackerel from Alaska, including Atlantic and Atka varieties, as these varieties are high in omega-3s but low in mercury. In contrast, king mackerel seems to have high mercury content. (33)

Sardines have been termed a "seafood superfood," as they are rich in omega-3s, selenium, vitamin D, calcium, and phosphorous, to name a few. They are also low in mercury. As an added bonus, they are one of the most sustainable fish available and are abundant in the oceans. This means that finding wild-caught sardines, while avoiding farmed sardines, is fairly easy.

Trout are an excellent source of omega-3s, vitamin B_6, vitamin B_{12}, selenium, and niacin. They also contain very little mercury.

Herring contains omega-3s, vitamin D, and selenium—all important cancer fighters. It is also rich in vitamin A, vitamin B_{12}, and potassium, selenium, and phosphorous. It is very low in mercury.

Tuna is another popular fish. It is an excellent source of omega-3 fatty acids as well as vitamins D, B_6, and B_{12}. It also contains iodine, potassium, and selenium. However, it is worth noting that tuna potentially contains higher levels of mercury, so pregnant women and young children should be careful. Interestingly, canned tuna contains less mercury than fresh tuna because the tuna used for canning tends to be smaller in size. However, due to mercury concerns, I don't rank tuna as highly as the other fish listed above in terms of health benefits.

Tilapia often shows up on restaurant menus, due to it tasting less "fishy" and also being relatively easy to obtain. However, it definitely isn't one of the healthier fish. Unfortunately, it is almost always farmed, meaning that it likely contains contaminants. Much of the tilapia produced today is genetically engineered. In addition, it contains a low amount of beneficial omega-3s and contains more omega-6s. We know that omega-6s are more prone to cause inflammation, and given the fact that most people already consume too many omega-6s, tilapia is only going to harm your ratio of omega-3 to omega-6.

When it comes to shellfish such as crabs, lobster, shrimp, oysters, and scallops, steer clear. They are "bottom feeders" that scavenge for waste products left over from other sea creatures. This means that they can contain high levels of harmful contaminants, including *E. coli* and hepatitis A. What's worse is that their uncomplicated digestive systems render them unable to expel waste. They also contain high levels of mercury. It's no wonder that shellfish cause so many allergic reactions!

As mentioned earlier, you don't have to eat seafood. If you do, opt for healthier options such as Alaskan salmon, Atlantic or Atka mackerel, sardines, trout, or herring. Choose wild-caught varieties. As with beef, chicken, or turkey, it doesn't need to be something you eat every day.

The Truth about Protein

There is so much confusion regarding protein. We know that protein is helpful for building muscle, and it also helps blunt the blood sugar impact of a high-carbohydrate meal. The supplement industry has long promoted protein powder as an essential supplement for athletes and people who are exercising regularly.

However, there is evidence that we consume too much protein today. Although we certainly want to make sure that we have enough protein, we also want to be careful not to eat too much. Thus, I recommend neither a high- or low-protein diet. You should simply get *enough* protein. We want to include enough protein in our diet to maintain a positive nitrogen balance, which is important for immune system function and maintaining muscle mass. Too much protein overloads the body, and getting more than is required simply isn't necessary to maintain optimal health. The amount of daily protein I recommend equates to one gram of protein for every kilogram of body weight (1 kg = 2.2 lbs.). Therefore, for a 180-pound person, this would equate to approximately 80 grams of protein daily.

When it comes to protein, most of us immediately think of red meat, poultry, fish, and dairy. Unfortunately, these foods are rich in the amino acid *methionine*. Methionine has been found to be a significant growth factor for cancer, dating back to research performed in the 1970s. (34) Additional research has confirmed cancer's dependence on methionine and suggested that restricting methionine could be a powerful tool to prevent and treat cancer. (35)

Research indicates that restricting methionine slows cancer growth in patients who have cancer. (36) There is also research supporting the idea that methionine restriction improves the effectiveness of chemotherapy. (37) For those who don't have cancer, it is possible that a low-methionine diet confers cancer prevention and life extension benefits. (38) Based on what we know about methionine, restricting it seems like a wise idea. The question is, by how much must we restrict it? We know that red meat, chicken, turkey, fish, eggs, and dairy have higher methionine content, while fruits, vegetables, beans, grains, nuts, and seeds have lower methionine content. Unfortunately, research has not yet evaluated a cutoff or threshold for methionine consumption (if it even exists).

If you have cancer, it is probably best to restrict methionine as much as possible. For many patients, this means eating exclusively plants and avoiding animal protein and seafood entirely. However, I cannot emphatically say that a piece of wild-caught salmon, grass-fed and grass-finished red meat, or organic free-range chicken a few times a week is detrimental to your health.

If you glean nothing else from this discussion on methionine, let it be that dietary methionine in high amounts seems to promote cancer growth. This doesn't mean that methionine is necessarily bad or that you shouldn't ever eat it. But it should give us pause when it comes to our dietary habits today, which rely so heavily on animal meats, dairy, and seafood.

The fact is, there is so much we still do not know about nutrition and cancer, and anyone who emphatically concludes that the science is settled on the topic is either misinformed or has an agenda to promote.

Organic vs. Conventional

As you have probably noticed, I am strongly in favor of organic food. I believe organic foods to be superior in quality for several reasons. Many harmful pesticides are forbidden from being used in organic foods. Often, these chemicals absorb into the food, making them impossible to simply wash off.

Organic foods, by definition, cannot be genetically modified. While many regulatory bodies insist on the safety of GMOs, there is no long-term evidence to support this. Remember, you can smoke for 20, 30, or 40 years before you are finally diagnosed with lung cancer. We simply cannot know what the long-term effects of consuming GMOs are. Shouldn't we err on the side of caution? As food purveyors are not required by law to disclose whether or not their foods are genetically modified, the USDA organic label is a guarantee that the food you are eating is not genetically modified.

Finally, organic animal products come from animals that have not been given hormones or antibiotics. While I do recommend reducing consumption of animal products, if and when you do enjoy them, I recommend enjoying organic varieties of dairy, meat, poultry, eggs, and fish.

References

(1) Kunzmann A.T., Coleman H.G., Huang W.Y., Berndt S.I. "The Association of Lifetime Alcohol Use with Mortality and Cancer Risk in Older Adults: A Cohort Study." *PLoS Med* 2018; 15(6): e1002585. doi: 10.1371/journal.pmed.1002585.

(2) Car Y., Willett W.C., Rimm E.B., et al. "Light to Moderate Intake of Alcohol, Drinking Patterns, and Risk of Cancer: Results from Two Prospective US Cohort Studies." *BMJ* 2015; 351: h4238.

(3) Fraser G.E., Jaceldo-Siegl K., Orlich M., et al. "Dairy, Soy, and Risk of Breast Cancer: Those Confounded Milks." *Int J Epidemiol* 2020; 49(5): 1526-37. doi: 10.1093/ije/dyaa007.

(4) Kroenke C.H., Kwan M.L., Sweeney C., et al. "High- and Low-Fat Dairy Intake, Recurrence, and Mortality after Breast Cancer Diagnosis." *J Natl Cancer Inst* 2013; 105(9): 616-23.

(5) Parodi P.W. "Dairy Product Consumption and the Risk of Breast Cancer." *J Am Coll Nutr* 2005; 24(6 Suppl): 556S-68S.

(6) Aune D., Rosenblatt D.A.N., Chan D.S.M., et al. "Dairy Products, Calcium, and Prostate Cancer Risk: A Systematic Review and Meta-Analysis of Cohort Studies." *Am J Clin Nutr* 2015; 101: 87-117. doi: 10.3945/ejcn.113.067157.

(7) Jeyaraman M.M., Abou-Setta A.M., Grant L., et al. "Dairy Product Consumption and Development of Cancer: An Overview of Reviews." *BMJ Open* 2019; 9:e023625. doi: 10.1136/bmjopen-2018-023625.

(8) Lampe J.W. "Dairy Products and Cancer." *J Am Coll Nutr* 2011; 30(5 Suppl 1): 464S-70S.

(9) Turner N.D., Lloyd S.K. "Association between Red Meat Consumption and Colon Cancer: A Systematic Review of Experimental Results." *Exp Biol Med (Maywood)* 2017; 242(8): 813-39. doi: 10.1177/1535370217693117.

(10) McAfee A.J., McSorley E.M., Cuskelly G.J., et al. "Red Meat from Animals Offered a Grass Diet Increases Plasma and Platelet n-3 PUFA in Healthy Consumers." *Br J Nutr* 2011; 105(1): 80-9. doi: 10.1017/S0007114510003090.

(11) Daley C.A., Abbott A., Doyle P.S., et al. "A Review of Fatty Acid Profiles and Antioxidant Content in Grass-Fed and Grain-Fed Beef." *Nutr J* 2010; 9: 10. doi: 10.1186/1475-2891-9-10.

(12) Zheng W., Lee S.A. "Well-Done Meat Intake, Heterocyclic Amine Exposure, and Cancer Risk." *Nutr Cancer* 2009; 61(4): 437-446. doi:10.1080/01635580802710741.

(13) Chiang V.S., Quek S.Y. "The Relationship of Red Meat with Cancer: Effects of Thermal Processing and Related Physiological Mechanisms." *Crit Rev Food Sci Nutr* 2017; 57(6): 1153-73. doi: 10.1080/10408398.2014.967833.

(14) Bouvard V., Loomis D., Guyton K.Z., et al; International Agency for Research on Cancer Monograph Working Group. "Carcinogenicity of Consumption of Red and Processed Meat." *Lancet Oncol* 2015; 16(16): 1599-600. doi: 10.1016/S1470-2045(15)00444-1.

(15) Shi Y., Yu P.W., Zeng D.Z. "Dose-Response Meta-Analysis of Poultry Intake and Colorectal Cancer Incidence and Mortality." *Eur J Nutr* 2015; 54(2): 243-50. doi: 10.1007/s00394-014-0705-0.

(16) Yang W.S., Wong M.Y., Vogtmann E., et al. "Meat Consumption and Risk of Lung Cancer: Evidence from Observational Studies." *Ann Oncol* 2012; 23(12): 3163-70. doi: 10.1093/annonc/mds207.

(17) Daniel C.R., Cross A.J., Graubard B.I., et al. "Prospective Investigation of Poultry and Fish Intake in Relation to Cancer Risk." *Cancer Prev Res* 2011; 4(11): 1903-11. doi: 10.1158/1940-6207.CAPR-11-0241.

(18) Richman E.L., Kenfield S.A., Stampfer M.J., et al. "Egg, Red Meat, and Poultry Intake and Risk of Lethal Prostate Cancer in the Prostate-Specific Antigen-Era: Incidence and Survival." *Cancer Prev Res (Phila)* 2011; 4(12): 2110-21. doi: 10.1158/1940-6207.CAPR-11-0354.

(19) Keum N., Lee D.H., Marchand N., et al. "Egg Intake and Cancers of the Breast, Ovary and Prostate: A Dose-Response Meta-Analysis of Prospective Observational Studies." *Br J Nutr* 2015; 114(7): 1099-107. doi: 10.1017/S0007114515002135.

(20) Tse G., Eslick G.D. "Egg Consumption and Risk of GI Neoplasms: Dose-Response Meta-Analysis and Systematic Review." *Eur J Nutr* 2014; 53(7): 1581-90. doi: 10.1007/s00394-014-0664-5.

(21) "What Is Aquaculture?" https://www.noaa.gov/stories/what-is-aquaculture. Accessed February 28, 2021.

(22) "EPA-FDA Advice about Eating Fish and Shellfish." https://www.epa.gov/fish-tech/epa-fda-advice-about-eating-fish-and-shellfish. Accessed February 28, 2021.

(23) Orlich M.J., Singh P.N., Sabate J., et al. "Vegetarian Dietary Patterns and the Risk of Colorectal Cancers." *JAMA Internal Med* 2015; 175(5): 767-76. doi: 10.1001/jamainternalmed.2015.59.

(24) Li N., Wu X., Xia L., et al. "Fish Consumption and Multiple Health Outcomes: Umbrella Review." *Trend Food Sci Tech* 2020; 99: 273-83. doi: 10.1016/j.tifs.2020.02.033.

(25) Song J., Su H., Wang B.L., et al. Fish Consumption and Lung Cancer Risk: Systematic Review and Meta-Analysis. *Nutr Cancer* 2014; 66: 539-49. doi: 10.1080/01635581.2014.894102.

(26) Liu Z.T., Lin A.H. "Dietary Factors and Thyroid Cancer Risk: A Meta-Analysis of Observational Studies. *Nutr Cancer* 2014; 66: 1165-78. doi: 10.1080/01635581.2014.951734.

(27) Stojanovic J., Giraldi L., Arzani D., et al. "Adherence to Mediterranean Diet and Risk of Gastric Cancer: Results of a Case-Control Study in Italy." *Eur J Cancer Prev* 2017; 26: 491-6. doi: 10.1097/CEJ.0000000000000371.

(28) Outzen M., Tjønneland A., Christensen J., Olsen A. "Fish Consumption and Prostate Cancer Risk and Mortality in a Danish Cohort Study." *Eur J Cancer Prev*. 2016 Nov 22. doi: 10.1097/CEJ.0000000000000330.

(29) Zhihui W., Weihua Y., Zupei W., Jinlin H. "Fish Consumption and Risk of Breast Cancer: Meta-Analysis of 27 Observational Studies." *Nutr Hosp* 2016; 33(3): 282. doi: 10.20960/nh.282.

(30) Hou R., Yao S.S., Liu J., et al. "Dietary n-3 Polyunsaturated Fatty Acids, Fish Consumption, and Endometrial Cancer Risk: A Meta-Analysis of Epidemiological Studies." *Oncotarget* 2017; 8(53): 91684-93. doi: 10.18632/oncotarget.18295.

(31) Jiang P.Y., Jiang Z.B., Shen K.X., Yue Y. "Fish Intake and Ovarian Cancer Risk: A Meta-Analysis of 15 Case-Control and Cohort Studies." *PLoS One* 2014; 9(4): e94601. doi: 10.1371/journal.pone.0094601.

(32) Foran J.A., Good D.H., Carpenter D.O., et al. "Quantitative Analysis of the Benefits and Risks of Consuming Farmed and Wild Salmon." *J Nutr* 2005; 135(11): 2639-43. doi: 10.1093/jn/135.11.263.

(33) "3 Healthiest (and Worst) Fish for Your Health. https://health.clevelandclinic.org/3-fish-you-should-love-and-3-fish-you-should-snub/. Accessed March 2, 2021.

(34) Halpern B.C., Clark B.R., Hardy D.N., et al. "The Effect of Replacement of Methionine by Homocysteine on Survival of Malignant and Normal Adult Mammalian Cells in Culture." *Proc Natl Acad Sci U S A* 1974; 71(4): 1133-6. doi: 10.1073/pnas.71.4.1133.

(35) Cellarier E., Durando X., Vasson M.P., et al. "Methionine Dependency and Cancer Treatment." *Cancer Treat Rev* 2003; 29(6): 489-99. doi: 10.1016/s0305-7372(03)00118-x.

(36) Cavuoto P., Fenech M.F. "A Review of Methionine Dependency and the Role of Methionine Restriction in Cancer Growth Control and Life-Span Extension." *Cancer Treat Rev* 2012; 38(6): 726-36. doi: 10.1016/j.ctrv.2012.01.004.

(37) Epner D.E. "Can Dietary Methionine Restriction Increase the Effectiveness of Chemotherapy in Treatment of Advanced Cancer?" *J Am Coll Nutr* 2001; 20(5 Suppl): 443S-449S; discussion 473S-475S. doi: 10.1080/07315724.2001.10719183.

(38) McCarty M.F, Barroso-Aranda J., Contreras F. "The Low-Methionine Content of Vegan Diets May Make Methionine Restriction Feasible as a Life Extension Strategy." *Med Hypotheses* 2009; 72(2): 125-8. doi: 10.1016/j.mehy.2008.07.044.

CHAPTER 8

Things You Should Minimize

There are some foods and food additives that I believe we should limit if we are to best utilize nutrition as a modality against cancer. Many of these foods are common in the Western diet.

Genetically Modified Organisms (GMOs)
Genetically modified organisms are living things that have had their genetic code changed in some way. Typically, DNA from one organism is added to another organism. The result is an animal, plant, virus, or bacteria that does not occur in nature; the goal of genetically modifying plants or animals used for food is to create products that are resistant to disease and more consistent in their flavor. From an agricultural profitability standpoint, this makes sense.

But what does this mean for our health? The Center for Food Safety has referred to the genetic engineering of plants and animals as "one of the greatest and most intractable environmental challenges of the 21st century." (1)

The Non-GMO Project considers corn, canola, soy, sugar beet, alfalfa, cotton, yellow summer squash, and zucchini as especially high-risk to our health. (2) Research shows that up to 92% of corn, 94% of soybeans, and 94% of cotton produced in the United States today is genetically engineered. (3) In addition, rice, tomatoes, and potatoes are also frequently genetically modified. (4)

The bigger problem with some of these GMOs is that they are often further processed into a variety of other ingredients that end up in many packaged products. In other words, a significant portion of our food supply today is genetically modified.

The reality is that we do not have long-term evidence confirming the safety of GMOs. In a way, it seems that purveyors of these products are using the mostly unsuspecting public as guinea pigs. It seems obvious that GMOs offer nothing of benefit to us and are likely capable of causing harm.

Avoiding GMOs should be a high priority for everyone. The best way to avoid genetically modified foods is to shop for organic varieties whenever possible. In the United States, the gold standard is the USDA Organic label. Foods that meet this standard cannot be genetically modified. Choose organic as much as possible.

If it's not organic, assume that it has some GMO components.

High-Glycemic Sweeteners

High-glycemic foods are any foods that cause a sharp rise in blood sugar levels—and thus, insulin—when they are consumed. These include high-fructose corn syrup, sugar, evaporated cane juice, brown rice syrup, or any other form of added sugar. Cancer cells, as we know, thrive on sugar.

Added sugar, in any form, is likely one of the most deleterious foods in the Western diet, in no small part because it is in virtually everything. Particularly if you eat processed foods or fast foods or drink sodas or any kind of sweetened beverage with regularity, you likely do not realize how much sugar you are consuming on a regular basis. We simply must become more mindful of how much sugar we consume and seek to minimize it if not eliminate it altogether.

Many patients ask if more "natural" sweeteners are okay, such as honey or agave. These are certainly healthier than white sugar, but they still cause a significant spike in blood glucose levels. Honey and agave should not be a staple in the diet, but are probably okay on occasion. Stevia is a better choice here, as it is also natural but essentially has no calories and little to no impact on blood sugar.

Heavily Processed Foods

The term *processed food* is a bit of a nebulous term, as it applies to any sort of food that has gone through any kind of process as part of its preparation. For example, ground beef—although it contains nothing but beef—is technically a processed food. For our purposes, we will consider most prepackaged foods as processed foods. These are foods that resemble nothing that comes directly from the earth: snack foods, crackers, chips, candy, frozen foods, and frozen precooked meals. If you have a hard time deciding which foods fit into this category, a good rule of thumb is to avoid anything with more than a few ingredients listed on the label, and certainly avoid anything with ingredients you do not recognize. Ideally, most of your foods should come without a list of ingredients.

There are several problems with the heavily processed foods that many people rely on for their nutrition. Often, these are high in sugar and/or refined carbohydrates. These often contain unnatural food additives, trans fats, preservatives, food dyes, GMOs, and high amounts of added sodium. Foods high in sodium should be avoided, because there is a link between a high-sodium diet and an increased risk of cancer. (5) Most preprepared food is usually much higher in sodium than many people realize.

Because we know that processed meats such as hot dogs, sausage, and pepperoni are not good for us, I recommend avoiding them entirely. However, if you must indulge, I recommend eating only organic varieties which do not contain any nitrates or nitrites. If you see ingredients such as sodium nitrite listed on the package, avoid it.

Shellfish

As we have already discussed, shellfish such as crabs, shrimp, lobster, oysters, scallops, and mussels are "bottom feeders" that scavenge for waste products left over from other sea-dwelling creatures. Their digestive systems make it more difficult for them to eliminate toxins. For these reasons, shellfish tend to have high levels of harmful contaminants such as bacteria, viruses, and mercury. I recommend avoiding shellfish altogether.

Trans Fats

Trans fats are man-made fats. They are created by adding hydrogen to certain oils, with the intention of prolonging the shelf life of processed foods. You can find trans fats in shortening and margarine, as well as a host of other pre-packaged foods. They are typically listed on the nutrition label as *hydrogenated* or *partially hydrogenated* oils.

For years, trans frats were promoted as being the safe alternative to animal fats. We have known for some time that trans fats actually increase the risk of heart disease rather than prevent it, and there is evidence now that they also increase the risk of cancer. (6, 7)

Trans fats should be avoided entirely. While most food purveyors have made a visible effort to remove trans fats from their food, these fats can still be found in certain processed foods. Please note that beneath a certain threshold, it is not necessary for purveyors to disclose the presence of trans fats in food. This is one more reason to avoid heavily processed foods entirely.

Be Mindful of How Your Food Is Cooked

I mentioned earlier that I do not recommend a fully raw diet and that cooking food is perfectly fine and, in many cases, beneficial. However, how your food is cooked is important to our discussion, because cooking in certain ways can introduce carcinogens into our food. Particularly, foods that have been fried run the risk of becoming carcinogenic. Any foods that have been charred, smoked, overcooked, or cooked at extremely high temperatures can also contain carcinogens. (8) Foods prepared in this way should be avoided, as well as any foods that have been burned.

Know What Is In Your Food

More than ever, it is necessary to be mindful about not just your food itself, but what might be contaminating your food. Unfortunately, there are a wide variety of food additives we should avoid. There are also substances that are simply byproducts of production and packaging that contaminate food.

Food Additives

Today, there exists a plethora of food additives that are not necessarily food themselves but serve some other purpose within food. These can be dyes, preservatives, or flavor enhancers. Many types of these food additives exist. Almost invariably, these ingredients are found in processed foods, which we should already be avoiding.

The list of these additives is quite long, and simply not enough evidence exists on each food additive to provide a comprehensive analysis of each one's effect on health. Regardless, the fact the we do not know the long-term effects of these substances seems to be some cause for concern. It is a prudent idea to avoid these as best we can, as they certainly are not necessary to include in a healthy diet.

There are some food additives, however, for which we do have evidence of a link to cancer and other health problems. I can confidently recommend avoiding the following.

BHA & BHT

Butylated hydroxyanisole (BHA) and butylated hydroxytoluene (BHT) are similar but unique preservatives often used in combination. Both are considered GRAS (generally recognized as safe) by the FDA. However, BHA is considered *reasonably anticipated to be carcinogenic to humans*, and BHT has been reported to trigger certain cancers in rats. Both are considered likely endocrine disruptors. (9)

Propylparaben

Propylparaben is commonly added to tortillas and muffins. It, too, is thought to be an endocrine disruptor and can influence genes important in breast cancers, accelerating growth in those cancer cells. (9)

Sodium Nitrite

Sodium nitrite has been known to be a cause of gastric cancers since the early part of the 20th century. In spite of this, it is still used in many types of cured meats, such as bacon, lunch meats, hot dogs, and sausages, as we discussed earlier.

Chemical Contaminants

In addition to additives that are put into our food purposefully, it is also important to be aware of some of the chemical contaminants inherent in our food supply. Some examples of these types of contaminants are substances such as mercury, cadmium, or other heavy metals known to contaminate fish, particularly fish higher in the food chain like tuna and swordfish. Most of us are aware that we should limit our intake of these foods in hopes of limiting our exposure to such chemicals. There are others that might be less well-known, which we should also be mindful of consuming.

Aflatoxin

Aflatoxins are metabolites of certain species of mold and fungi which can infest crops, including corn, peanuts, and cottonseed. They are also known to contaminate dairy products, eggs, nuts, almonds, and certain spices. These are among the most carcinogenic, naturally-occurring substances on earth. Aflatoxins have been linked to liver cancer and other health problems in humans. (10)

Bisphenol A (BPA)

BPA is found in the polycarbonate and plastic packaging used in many kinds of food; it is also present in plastic ware, plastic cups, and other plastic products commonly found in the kitchen. Often, aluminum cans are lined with plastic that contains BPA. BPA can leach into food and beverages when plastic becomes too hot, too cold, scratched, or otherwise damaged.

While the FDA claims that the amount of BPA found in food is likely not harmful (11), other research suggests that BPA might play a role in cancer development. (12) BPA is an endocrine disruptor, and as such, it might have the ability to influence hormone-dependent cancers like breast and prostate cancers.

Gluten

Gluten is a protein found in wheat that poses no risk to most people. However, for those with celiac disease, gluten stimulates the body's immune system to attack its own cells, causing damage in the intestines which can lead to cancer. (13) These individuals must avoid gluten entirely.

Interestingly, there exists another group of people who aren't allergic to gluten but who are sensitive to it. This is termed *gluten sensitivity*. When gluten sensitivity exists, consuming gluten might cause non-specific gastrointestinal symptoms such as abdominal pain, cramping, and loose stools. It can also cause other symptoms, such as fatigue and headaches. The cancer risk in gluten-sensitive patients has not been established, but it seems that these individuals should also exclude gluten from their diets as much as possible.

For these individuals, there are other healthy grains that do not contain gluten and can be safely consumed. These include oats, quinoa, amaranth, and buckwheat. Sprouted grains and ancient grains are often acceptable options for those who are gluten sensitive.

Be wary of products labeled gluten-free, as not all are necessarily healthy. Many contain some unhealthy ingredients.

Glyphosate

Many people know glyphosate by its brand name, Roundup, which is manufactured by the Monsanto company. Glyphosate is the most heavily-used pesticide ever produced. Genetically modified organisms (GMOs) are frequently genetically engineered for the sole purpose of being able to withstand high amounts of pesticides such as glyphosate.

For years, we were told it was safe. Today, we know that glyphosate is carcinogenic. (14) While the risk is highest for farmers who regularly handle glyphosate, this pesticide is something we should seek to eliminate from our diets. You can largely eliminate the risk of your food being contaminated with glyphosate by shopping for organic products.

rBGH

Recombinant bovine growth hormone (rBGH) is also known as recombinant bovine somatotropin (rBST). This synthetic form of bovine growth hormone is used to increase milk production in cows. Dairy products from cows treated with rBGH are often tainted with both these hormones and insulin-like growth factor 1 (IGF-1), a hormone known to influence cancer growth. (15) Despite the fact that Europe, Canada, and other parts of the world have banned the use of these hormones, the United States continues to allow their use.

References

(1) "About Genetically Engineered Foods" http://www.centerforfoodsafety.org/issues/311/ge-foods/about-ge-foods. Accessed March 13, 2021.

(2) "What is a GMO?" https://www.nongmoproject.org/gmo-facts/what-is-gmo/. Accessed March 13, 2021.

(3) "Recent Trends in GE Adoption" https://www.ers.usda.gov/data-products/adoption-of-genetically-engineered-crops-in-the-us/recent-trends-in-ge-adoption.aspx. Accessed March 13, 2021.

(4) Bhatia, MD Dr. Tasneem. "10 Most Common GMO Foods To Avoid." *FOOD MATTERS®*, Food Matters, 19 Nov. 2017, www.foodmatters.com/article/10-most-common-gmo-foods.

(5) Wang, Xiao-Qin, et al. "Review of Salt Consumption and Stomach Cancer Risk: Epidemiological and Biological Evidence." *World Journal of Gastroenterology*, vol. 15, no. 18, 2009, p. 2204., doi:10.3748/wjg.15.2204.

(6) "Trans Fats May Increase Risk." Breastcancer.org, www.breastcancer.org/research-news/20080411b.

(7) Slattery, Martha L., et al. "Trans-Fatty Acids and Colon Cancer." *Nutrition and Cancer*, vol. 39, no. 2, 2001, pp. 170–175., doi:10.1207/s15327914nc392_2.

(8) "Chemicals in Meat Cooked at High Temperatures and Cancer Risk." *National Cancer Institute*, www.cancer.gov/about-cancer/causes-prevention/risk/diet/cooked-meats-fact-sheet.

(9) "Generally Recognized as Safe – But Is It?" *EWG*, Nov. 2014, www.ewg.org/research/ewg-s-dirty-dozen-guide-food-additives/generally-recognized-as-safe-but-is-it#.Wl6Oj62ZORs.

(10) "Department of Animal Science - Plants Poisonous to Livestock." *Cornell University Department of Animal Science*, poisonousplants.ansci.cornell.edu/toxicagents/aflatoxin/aflatoxin.html.

(11) Center for Food Safety and Applied Nutrition. "Public Health Focus - Bisphenol A (BPA): Use in Food Contact Application." US Food and Drug Administration Home Page, Center for Food Safety and Applied Nutrition, www.fda.gov/newsevents/publichealthfocus/ucm064437.htm#summary.

(12) Stern, Victoria. "Does BPA Increase Cancer Risk?" *Medscape*, 4 Mar. 2015, www.medscape.com/viewarticle/840559.

(13) Freeman, Hugh James. "Malignancy in Adult Celiac Disease." *World Journal of Gastroenterology*, vol. 15, no. 13, 2009, p. 1581., doi:10.3748/wjg.15.1581.

(14) "Known and Probable Human Carcinogens." *American Cancer Society*, www.cancer.org/cancer/cancer-causes/general-info/known-and-probable-human-carcinogens.html.

(15) "About rBGH." Center for Food Safety, www.centerforfoodsafety.org/issues/1044/rbgh/about-rbgh.

CHAPTER 9

How to Fast

Incorporating Fasting into Your Life

I believe that we have made a good case for the benefits of fasting, particularly as it relates to fasting's utility against cancer. I have also outlined how nutrition can best be utilized as a modality to both fight and prevent cancer according to the best research we currently have available. So, we have a good idea about *how* to eat in order to fight cancer. Fasting, however, is all about *when* you eat. So while we know that fasting might confer tremendous benefit, we must discuss the variety of ways you can safely and effectively incorporate fasting into your lifestyle to maximize both your health and your defense against cancer.

Fasting as a tool is really quite simple; it means you don't eat for a specified period of time. Fasting is unique as a dietary tool in this regard, as "diets" will have you restrict certain foods, potentially interfering with your normal life. Simply abstaining from eating, however, is much easier to integrate and has nothing to do with what you might eat during your eating window, necessarily.

How you incorporate fasting into your life is more nuanced than just not eating for random or indefinite periods of time. In reality, there are a variety of ways we can strategically incorporate fasting into our lives to reap a myriad of benefits. Fasting is something that has been practiced for millennia, and certainly, in prehistoric times, our ancestors would have necessarily endured periods of fasting punctuated by periods of feasting. Fasting is very much woven into our DNA, even if modern life has largely eliminated the circumstances which would make fasting a necessity. In most Western cultures, fasting as a regular cultural or religious practice has virtually been eliminated. So while it might take some time to adjust to fasting, it is certainly not without biological precedent for humans. After a period of adjustment, you will likely find that you feel much better than you did before you incorporated fasting.

Fasting does require a certain amount of conditioning, and this is particularly true with some of the more intense fasting strategies we will discuss. Therefore, I encourage you to tread carefully. With longer fasts especially, there are associated risks, particularly if you have never fasted before, which is why I encourage you to talk with your physician before implementing fasting. This is even more important if you take medications or if you are dealing with certain health problems, cancer included. It is imperative to learn about the different kinds of fasting protocols and then tailor their use to your particular health goals.

Furthermore, I will stop short of recommending a one-size-fits-all approach to fasting as a health strategy. Studies examining the benefits of fasting are still emerging, and our knowledge about its utility as a health protocol is still in its infancy. However, as we have seen, we know there is *something* there, and the preliminary research which has been done leads me to believe that fasting does facilitate some powerful functions within the body that we stand to benefit from, particularly regarding cancer.

That said, fasting is not a panacea or a cure-all, much in the same way that nutrition is neither of those things. Fasting (and nutrition) are merely two strategies that should be used as part of a unilateral approach to facilitating great health and preventing disease. In other words, I would never recommend that someone fast without also recommending they quit smoking cigarettes—fasting will not save you from the risk posed by smoking! This might seem like common sense to some people, but in a world rife with misinformation, particularly when it comes to information about cancer and so-called "natural" or "alternative" ways to combat it, it bears repeating that there is no silver bullet and common sense still applies. That, however, does not mean that strategies such as fasting do not confer serious benefits or have no utility when done in an appropriate way. I believe quite the opposite to be true.

So as we proceed through this chapter, keep in mind I am merely presenting the most common methods of integrating fasting into your lifestyle—not recommending one fasting regimen in particular. I will emphasize what the research says about particular kinds of fasts where appropriate. I recommend starting small, usually with short-term fasts, which we will discuss first. After you have some experience with these types of fasts, you may want to try longer fasts, which can confer benefits beyond what short-term fasts can provide. I will also discuss the risks these types of fasts can pose so that you can confidently proceed with an understanding of those risks and how to mitigate them. It bears repeating, however, that there are examples in the literature of people going for over a year without eating (with some vitamin/mineral supplementation and under the watchful eye of physicians, of course!). While such an extreme fast is obviously unnecessary for most people, it does underscore the fact that long-term fasting can be done safely and effectively when executed properly.

How to Fast

First, let's reiterate what fasting means. Technically speaking, *fasting* means "consuming no calories." In practice, this requires the consumption of non-caloric drinks only. The types of beverages that are permitted on a fast include water, black coffee, and tea—all unsweetened and without milk or cream.

While there are some types of fasts that recommend forgoing water, there is absolutely no therapeutic benefit to this. On the contrary, it is vitally important to stay hydrated while you are fasting. Many of the negative side effects of fasting, such as headaches, stem from dehydration. Water is not only permitted, but it is encouraged. I generally recommend that patients strive to drink half of their body weight in ounces. However, while fasting, the amount of water needed might be higher than this. Fasting lowers insulin, which prompts the release of fluid from the body in the form of urine. You may find yourself using the bathroom more frequently during a fast. It is vital to replenish those lost fluids so you do not get dehydrated.

Black coffee and tea both contain no calories and are permitted while fasting. Coffee and some types of tea contain caffeine, which is an appetite suppressant and may be beneficial when starting out on a fasting protocol. Herbal teas are permitted, as well as traditional tea brewed from tea leaves. Adding small amounts of herbs or spices, such cinnamon, is permitted as well. Coffee and tea should not be consumed exclusively in lieu of water.

Zero-Calorie Sweeteners
While sugar, honey, agave, and other sweeteners are certainly off-limits while you are fasting, zero-calorie sweeteners, such as aspartame, sucralose, and stevia, do technically qualify as permissible when fasting. Stevia is a sweetener derived from an herb, while sucralose and aspartame are both sugar substitutes that are commonly found in diet beverages and other diet sweets. The general consensus is that none of these sweeteners will spike your insulin or blood sugar levels, although there is some evidence that this might not be the case with sugar substitutes. (1) There are other reasons to avoid sugar substitutes, including the fact that they might contribute to insulin resistance, weight gain, and even cancer, although some research points to the contrary. (2, 3) Generally, I recommend avoiding artificial sweeteners such as sucralose and aspartame. If you must sweeten your coffee or tea, opt for organic stevia products.

Electrolytes
Electrolytes include substances such as sodium, magnesium, and potassium, and these minerals are an important aspect of hydration. Together with the kidneys, electrolytes help our bodies maintain a proper amount of fluid, as well as facilitate a number of other important biological processes. However, when we fast and our bodies begin to release fluid in the form of urine, stool, and sweat, some of these electrolytes can get flushed out as well. The most common symptom of electrolyte imbalance is headache. Longer-term fasts that are not

properly executed run the risk of more significant complications due to electrolyte imbalance. To that end, it may be beneficial to supplement with electrolytes while you are fasting. This is a strategy that is more important on longer-term fasts, so if you are merely doing intermittent fasting, supplementing with electrolytes is likely unnecessary. However, there are high-quality electrolyte replacement powders that contain no calories, are naturally flavored, and use stevia as a sweetener. I recommend keeping some on hand, just in case you find yourself needing repletion during your fast.

Juice Fasts Are a Misnomer

Juice fasts, though they are a popular health trend, do not really constitute a true fast. Even freshly squeezed juices contain calories and are often high in sugar, which will raise your insulin, largely defeating the purpose of the fast. The same goes for vegetable juices. This is not to say that these are not healthy or abundant in nutrition—they are. However, these should be relegated to your eating window and avoided during the fasting window. The only time I recommend juice fasts are when people have difficulty conducting a true fast, and these situations are rare.

Fat Fasting, Bone Broth

Fat fasting involves including tiny bits of pure fat, such as cream, butter, olive oil, etc., during your fasting window. The purported benefits of fat fasting are the mitigation of hunger during a fast, and some people report better concentration. This is something Dr. Jason Fung—an authority on the benefits of fasting—discusses, along with adding small amounts of bone broth, or foods that are mostly fat with negligible carbohydrates or protein, such as walnuts, macadamia nuts, etc. The idea is that these foods can help you maintain fasting for longer periods. (4) In the case of longer fasts, these strategies might be beneficial. For shorter fasts, they are likely unnecessary. Plus, it can be easy to over-indulge, thus mitigating the effects of fasting.

Intermittent Fasting (IF)

The first type of fasting we will discuss is a form of short-term fasting called *intermittent fasting*. It is very likely that you have heard of intermittent fasting, as it has become one of the most popular fasting strategies in recent years. Intermittent fasting is easy to incorporate into your regimen, yet the health benefits can be profound.

In some sense, we all participate in this kind of fasting, because most of us do not wake up in the middle of the night to eat. Chances are, you are already technically fasting for about 10–12 hours a day. In that sense, incorporating intermittent fasting into your life is as easy as extending that period of not eating—your fasting window—a few more hours on a daily basis.

All of these regimens are routines you can follow on a daily basis.

16:8

The 16:8 method is one of the most common methods of incorporating intermittent fasting into your regimen. The 16:8 method involves fasting for 16 hours a day, leaving an 8-hour eating window. It can be as simple as skipping breakfast, eating lunch at noon, and finishing dinner by 8:00 p.m. You can structure your meals however you like during those 8 hours as long as you are abstaining from any caloric consumption during the 16-hour fasting window.

This is really one of the easiest ways to incorporate fasting into your regimen. But can something as simple as skipping one meal really elicit profound results? Interestingly, research indicates that intermittent fasting might be beneficial for weight loss and obesity reduction. (5, 6) Other research indicates that intermittent fasting can lower the risk of type 2 diabetes. (7) Intermittent fasting might also be beneficial in lowering blood pressure in obese adults. (8) Intermittent fasting might protect brain health and memory while slowing diseases that affect the brain. (10) And, a review of studies in 2017 found that intermittent fasting reduces the risk of non-alcoholic fatty liver disease and cancer. (10)

All of these benefits can be attributed to simply restricting your eating window to 8 hours a day. How difficult is it to merely skip breakfast or dinner on a daily basis? It is true that many people are accustomed to eating whenever they wish throughout the day, and changing these habits can be difficult. Invariably, changing your eating schedule will require some adjustment, but the 16:8 method of fasting is so simple, so risk-free, and so low impact that it is really a no-brainer for most people to implement. It is also a great way to introduce yourself to fasting.

20:4 and OMAD

The 20:4 method of fasting involves extending your fasting window to 20 hours a day with a 4-hour feeding window. This is a natural extension of the 16:8 fasting method. This method of IF was popularized in the book *The Warrior Diet* by Ori Hofmekler.

According to cancer researcher Dr. Thomas Seyfried, all fasting is beneficial. (4) The longer you can extend your fast (within reason), the more of those benefits you are likely to enjoy. This underscores the way fasting is interwoven into our genetic makeup—our bodies are designed to endure periods of fasting, and even thrive under those conditions.

For most people, jumping into a 20:4 fasting regimen would be tough, but after a period of time on a 16:8 regimen, you might find that you can make the jump to 20:4. You will likely see that the longer you go without eating, the more mental clarity, focus, and energy you have throughout the day. On a 20:4 regimen, for example, you might break your fast at 3:00 p.m. every day with a protein shake or a snack, and then finish eating dinner by 7:00 p.m.

The final logical extension of intermittent fasting is one meal a day, or OMAD for short. With OMAD, you would pick one meal, whether it is breakfast, lunch, or dinner, and eat that meal at the same time every day. OMAD extends the fasting window to around 23–24 hours daily. With OMAD, the one meal needs to be a large, highly nutritious meal. The desire to binge on unhealthy food will need to be controlled.

Intermittent fasting is beneficial for a few reasons. First, it is easy to implement into your lifestyle. You can still enjoy family meals, special occasions, and the so-called joy of the feast. Second, intermittent fasting does not necessarily encourage calorie counting or dictate what you can eat during the fasting window. You should, however, focus on nutrition during your eating window. Nutritious, whole foods, like vegetables, fruits, nuts, and whole grains should be your focus. And third, with intermittent fasting, you can still meet all of your nutritional needs and avoid malnutrition.

However, consistency is key. Starting with a 16:8 regimen for a period of time is a good way to ease into fasting as a lifestyle. By taking this small step, you will be taking advantage of lowered insulin levels, increased levels of growth hormone, better metabolism, better focus, more energy, and improved mental clarity.

What Happens if I Get Hungry?

Intermittent fasting is a good introduction to structuring the times of day at which you eat. However, as with any habit, fasting takes time to feel natural. In the beginning, you will undoubtedly feel hungry. Now is a good time to talk about hunger and what that feeling really means.

Intuitively, we tend to assume that we feel hunger when our stomach is empty and our body needs food for fuel. However, research into circadian rhythms shows that hunger for most people is lowest in the morning—often 10 to 14 hours after your last meal. So it is not just an empty stomach that drives hunger. In reality, hunger is a hormonal signal—our brain telling us to eat—which has many triggers and is highly sensitive to how we program it.

Think about it: do you ever smell fresh bread baking, smell breakfast being prepared, or hear steaks sizzling on the grill and start to feel the gnawing of hunger pangs? These sensory inputs can easily trigger hunger. Simply seeing food on a television commercial can even initiate hunger. These signals are *not* your body communicating a true need to eat.

Furthermore, if you are accustomed to eating at certain times every day, your body is programmed to expect food at those specific times. Chances are good that around lunch every day, you start feeling your stomach growl. Similarly, if you are accustomed to snacking throughout the day, you might experience hunger much of the time. These are hormonal signals that we have trained our bodies to communicate, telling us to eat.

We also tend to eat for a variety of reasons. We eat when we are bored, sad, celebrating, and attending social gatherings. All of these situations can be triggers to eat.

It is important to remember that hunger is not necessarily a signal that you *must* eat. It is important to remember that hunger comes in waves, and if you can ride out a bout of hunger, it will dissipate. Often, people on extended fasts do not report hunger pangs after about the second day. Some researchers speculate that this is due to the body being fueled by ketones, or by metabolized fat, which may act as a natural hunger suppressant.

While you are acclimating to intermittent fasting, chances are you will be hungry for the first couple of days during your fasting window. Once you program your body to expect food at a certain time, you will likely find that your hunger patterns change in relation to your eating patterns.

While you will certainly experience hunger, particularly in the beginning, you should never feel *sick* or *bad* while fasting. If you start to feel poorly, with symptoms such as nausea, dizziness, or headache, you should break your fast.

Weekly Structured Fasting

Some fasting strategies focus on the way you eat for an entire week instead of focusing on what you eat daily. For some people, this can be a good strategy, because it allows for days of so-called normal eating schedules. You will still glean the benefits of fasting while also enjoying days of not structuring your eating. These are slightly more advanced strategies than intermittent fasting, since they involve longer periods without food.

Not every strategy is right for every person. It may take some time to understand which fasting strategy has the most benefit for you and helps you achieve your health goals.

Fasting One Day a Week

Fasting one day a week involves one 24-hour fast per week. This is as simple as fasting from dinner on day one to dinner on day two, then having a normal eating schedule for the rest of the week.

Single 24-hour fasts are very easy to incorporate into your lifestyle. This is similar to OMAD fasting, which is essentially a 23-hour fast every day. Fasting one day a week is likely best paired with intermittent fasting. A good schedule with this sort of fasting could be as follows:

> **Monday–Saturday:** 16:8 intermittent fasting (final meal is dinner on Saturday night)
> **Sunday:** Dinner only

This allows you to glean the benefits of intermittent fasting while still getting the benefits of a slightly extended fast. This can be a good strategy working into OMAD fasting.

2:5

The 2:5 method is another simple way of structuring your eating throughout the week. This involves two non-consecutive days per week of 24-hour fasting, with a "normal" eating structure on all other days of the week. Incorporating this method of fasting is as easy as picking two days a week during which you would only eat dinner. This can be a good strategy for those trying to lose weight.

A schedule on a 2:5 fasting regimen might look like this:

> **Monday:** Unstructured eating, or 16:8 intermittent fasting
> **Tuesday:** Unstructured eating, or 16:8 intermittent fasting
> **Wednesday:** Dinner only
> **Thursday:** Unstructured eating, or 16:8 intermittent fasting
> **Friday:** Unstructured eating, or 16:8 intermittent fasting
> **Saturday:** Unstructured eating, or 16:8 intermittent fasting
> **Sunday:** Dinner only

A popular modification of the 2:5 fasting schedule involves only eating 500–600 calories on fasting days.

3:4

A 3:4 fasting schedule is the natural extension of the 2:5 fasting schedule and involves adding another day of 24-hour fasting to your weekly regimen. A week on the 3:4 fasting schedule might look like this:

> **Monday:** Unstructured eating, or 16:8 intermittent fasting
> **Tuesday:** Dinner only

> **Wednesday:** Unstructured eating, or 16:8 intermittent fasting
> **Thursday:** Dinner only
> **Friday:** Unstructured eating, or 16:8 intermittent fasting
> **Saturday:** Dinner only
> **Sunday:** Unstructured eating, or 16:8 intermittent fasting

Once you become accustomed to eating on a 2:5 schedule, it is likely very easy to progress to the 3:4 schedule. All of these can be used to ultimately work up to OMAD if desired. Similar to the 5:2 fasting schedule, an alternate version allows for eating only 500–600 calories on fasting days.

Alternate-Day Fasting

Alternate-day fasting is the most intense weekly structured fasting regimen because it involves multiple 36-hour fasts per week. With alternate-day fasting, you eat "normally" every other day while eating nothing the following day. An alternate-day fasting schedule might look something like this:

> **Monday:** Breakfast 8:00 a.m., final meal finished by 8:00 p.m.
> **Tuesday:** Fast
> **Wednesday:** Breakfast 8:00 a.m., final meal finished by 8:00 p.m.
> **Thursday:** Fast

Friday: Breakfast 8:00 a.m., final meal finished by 8:00 p.m.
Saturday: Fast
Sunday: Breakfast 8:00 a.m., final meal finished by 8:00 p.m.
Monday: Fast
Tuesday: Breakfast 8:00 a.m., final meal finished by 8:00 p.m.
Wednesday: Fast
Thursday: Breakfast 8:00 a.m., final meal finished by 8:00 p.m.
Friday: Fast
Saturday: Breakfast 8:00 a.m., final meal finished by 8:00 p.m.
Sunday: Fast
(Repeat)

There is a modified version of alternate-day fasting wherein you consume between 500 and 600 calories per day on fast days. This does not constitute a true fast and is more akin to a fasting-mimicking diet. Given how difficult alternate-day fasting can be, this might be a good strategy for many people. You will still glean many of the same benefits, and many practitioners use this method with good results.

Interestingly, there is some good research when it comes to alternate-day fasting and its health benefits. A clinical trial in 2019 found that alternate-day fasting might be more effective than traditional dieting for losing weight, controlling blood sugar, and lowering blood sugar. (11) The American Journal of Medicine published research that found that alternate-day fasting may reduce the risk of heart disease. They concluded this was because alternate-day fasting reduces blood pressure, helps control weight and cholesterol, and reduces blood sugar levels. (12)

Finally, alternate-day fasting has been observed to slow tumor progression in patients undergoing cancer treatment. (13)

Binge Eating, Cravings, and Fasting

While fasting is a healthy and beneficial protocol for most people to incorporate, some people do have concerns about food cravings as well as binge eating following a fast.

It is worth reiterating that fasting is *not* an eating disorder. Of course, eating too little (anorexia) is an eating disorder. Even though you are incorporating periods of not eating into your life, you should still eat plenty of calories during your eating window! Part of the joy of fasting is enjoying the periods of feasting that break the fast. This is partly why I have included so much information on nutrition in this book. When you break your fast, you should focus on whole, minimally processed, highly nutritious foods. When fasting, please keep your nutritional needs in mind, including how much protein and total calories you need, what your fiber requirements are, etc. Fasting *does not* mean you should be creating nutritional deficiencies.

However, it is important to make sure you do not go beyond those needs. Certainly, there is some risk of overindulging when you break a fast—this has far less to do with the needs of your body and far more to do with psychology. This underscores the necessity and utility of cultivating mindfulness about what we eat. Do you frequently eat beyond being merely satisfied, to the point that you are uncomfortably full? It is important to learn to pay attention to your body's satiety signals. Ultimately, you should map that onto your daily nutritional needs and learn how those two things can exist in harmony. Interestingly, people who fast typically find themselves satiated with much less food than they were previously accustomed to eating.

Similarly, food cravings are merely psychological. Do you really *need* the box of donuts? Nutritionally, the answer is no. Have you conditioned your body to expect junk foods, unhealthy fats, lots of sugar, or salt? Given the standard American diet, the answer for many people is likely yes. One of the benefits of fasting is breaking the cycle of merely giving into any craving or hunger that might arise. Fasting is a good way to begin cultivating mindfulness about what we put in our mouths and the effects that foods can have on our bodies, reminding us that we are in control of what we provide our bodies for nourishment.

Extended Fasting

Anything beyond 42 hours is considered an extended fast. The idea of going nearly two entire days without any food whatsoever seems foreign to most people, but it is important to remember that people have participated in extended fasts for millennia as part of religious observance with no reported ill effects. Jesus fasted in the desert for 40 days. Extended fasts simply are not as unusual as they may seem.

That said, extended fasts are likely not something you should try if you have not experimented successfully with intermittent fasting and some of the longer periods of fasting. Extended fasts are something you should discuss with your doctor, particularly if you are diabetic or taking certain medications. The risks associated with fasting increase as the duration increases. However, this does not mean that longer-term fasts are necessarily dangerous or without use. On the contrary, extended fasts—when executed in a safe, proper way—might have some profound benefits, particularly related to cancer.

Fasting 48 Hours and Beyond
Extended fasts usually last between 2 and 14 days. A full 48-hour fast could look like eating dinner on Monday evening and not eating again until dinner Wednesday evening. A full 48-hour fast does not come with serious risk, provided you are staying hydrated. Interestingly though, day 2 is typically the toughest day for those on a fasting regimen. Pushing through the 2-day mark, whether you have experience with fasting or not, is typically the hardest barrier to cross. Most people experience relief from hunger, which coincides with the hunger hormone ghrelin decreasing. In addition, day three is also associated with increased mental clarity, abundant energy, and a feeling of euphoria.

Therefore, many practitioners suggest that if you can make it two days, pushing through to a 5, 7, or even 14-day fast is not nearly as difficult as many would assume. And interestingly, this is where we begin to see a notable increase in many of the associated benefits of fasting.

It is worth reviewing a timeline of what happens in the body when we fast:

Day 1
The body is primarily fueled by glycogen in the liver. As glycogen levels become depleted, the body begins the process of gluconeogenesis, which provides fuel as glycogen levels run out.

Day 2
The body enters a state of ketosis. This is the process wherein fat reserves are broken down for fuel. Notably, some of the beneficial aspects of fasting begin to accelerate: human growth hormone increases, cellular autophagy increases, and the body's hormonal response becomes more efficient (e.g., cells become more sensitive to insulin). (14)

Day 3
Many of the side effects of fasting, such as fatigue, brain fog, lethargy, and hunger, begin to dissipate. Ketone levels continue to increase.

Day 4
Approximately 75% of the brain's energy is derived from ketone bodies at this point. Autophagy begins to reach peak levels.

Day 5
Many of the fasting benefits begin to reach their maximum levels. Autophagy and HGH are at peak levels.

Still, some practitioners use fasts lasting between 7 and 14 days. Dr. Jason Fung uses fasts lasting between one and two weeks with patients suffering from severe type 2 diabetes in his practice. (4) Fasts of this duration likely require some supervision, particularly if you have health problems. Supplementation with electrolytes and some micronutrients will also likely be necessary. While there can be profound benefits for fasting beyond 5 days—and we know there is no set cap on how long a person can fast (given enough fat reserves)—the risk of complications increases the longer the fast is continued.

Frequency of Extended Fasting

Obviously, extended fasting is not a practice to use on a weekly basis. The frequency with which you should engage in extended fasting is largely dependent on your goals. If you have significant weight to lose, extended fasts of 4–5 days could ostensibly be done once a month, with intermittent fasting used between the extended fasts. This is a significant modality for losing excess weight, which is very beneficial in lowering your risk for getting cancer. If you have a healthy BMI, extended fasts once a quarter may be more appropriate. You will still glean the notable benefits of the extended fasts without affecting your lean muscle mass. Some of these effects likely have anticancer benefits.

Know the Risks

One of the biggest risks of extended fasting is the risk of *refeeding syndrome*. Refeeding syndrome most often occurs in people who are severely malnourished, and those most at risk for this phenomenon are people with anorexia, alcoholism, and extremely low body weight.

Refeeding syndrome occurs during the first two days of breaking a fast and is the result of depleted electrolytes, particularly phosphorus. As you begin to consume food again, insulin levels rise, promoting the synthesis of glycogen, protein, and fat. These processes require minerals, and if those stores of minerals are already depleted, muscle tissue can begin to break down, including the muscles comprising the heart and the diaphragm. Depletion of electrolytes such as potassium and magnesium can cause abnormal heart rhythms, breathing difficulty, and cardiac arrest.

Thankfully, refeeding syndrome is exceedingly rare. The biggest risk factor is malnutrition, and it generally only occurs in people who have been deprived of food for long periods of time against their will. In addition, your body is adept at hanging on to electrolytes. The kidneys work to keep these minerals in balance even in the absence of food. That said, supplementing with electrolytes is a common technique for those on extended fasts and might help mitigate the less severe side affects associated with fasting, such as headaches.

Ultimately, however, if you are malnourished to the point that you have experienced wasting or cachexia, extended fasts may not be a safe strategy for you to employ.

References

(1) Tandel, Kirtida R. "Sugar Substitutes: Health Controversy over Perceived Benefits." *Journal of Pharmacology and Pharmacotherapeutics*, vol. 2, no. 4, 2011, pp. 236–243., https://doi.org/10.4103/0976-500x.85936.

(2) Rubin, Rita. "Could Artificial Sweeteners Raise Your Blood Sugar?" *WebMD*, WebMD, 18 Sept. 2014, https://www.webmd.com/diet/news/20140917/artificial-sweeteners-blood-sugar.

(3) Nagpure, Shailesh, et al. "Effect of Artificial Sweeteners on Insulin Resistance among Type-2 Diabetes Mellitus Patients." *Journal of Family Medicine and Primary Care*, vol. 9, no. 1, 2020, p. 69., https://doi.org/10.4103/jfmpc.jfmpc_329_19.

(4) Fung, J., & Moore, J. (2016). *The Complete Guide to Fasting: Heal Your Body through Intermittent, Alternate-Day, and Extended Fasting*. Victory Belt Publishing.

(5) Byrne, N M, et al. "Intermittent Energy Restriction Improves Weight Loss Efficiency in Obese Men: The Matador Study." *International Journal of Obesity*, vol. 42, no. 2, 2017, pp. 129–138., https://doi.org/10.1038/ijo.2017.206.

(6) Moro, Tatiana, et al. "Effects of Eight Weeks of Time-Restricted Feeding (16/8) on Basal Metabolism, Maximal Strength, Body Composition, Inflammation, and Cardiovascular Risk Factors in Resistance-Trained Males." *Journal of Translational Medicine*, vol. 14, no. 1, 2016, https://doi.org/10.1186/s12967-016-1044-0.

(7) Barnosky, Adrienne R., et al. "Intermittent Fasting vs. Daily Calorie Restriction for Type 2 Diabetes Prevention: A Review of Human Findings." *Translational Research*, vol. 164, no. 4, 2014, pp. 302–311., https://doi.org/10.1016/j.trsl.2014.05.013.

(8) Gabel, Kelsey, et al. "Effects of 8-Hour Time Restricted Feeding on Body Weight and Metabolic Disease Risk Factors in Obese Adults: A Pilot Study." *Nutrition and Healthy Aging*, vol. 4, no. 4, 2018, pp. 345–353., https://doi.org/10.3233/nha-170036.

(9) Collier, Roger. "Intermittent Fasting: The Science of Going Without." *Canadian Medical Association Journal*, vol. 185, no. 9, 2013, https://doi.org/10.1503/cmaj.109-4451.

(10) Patterson, Ruth E., and Dorothy D. Sears. "Metabolic Effects of Intermittent Fasting." *Annual Review of Nutrition*, vol. 37, no. 1, 2017, pp. 371–393., https://doi.org/10.1146/annurev-nutr-071816-064634.

(11) Dong T.A., Sandesara P.B., Dhindsa D.S., et al. "Intermittent Fasting: A Heart Healthy Dietary Pattern?" *Am J Med.* 2020; PMID: 32330491

(12) Parvaresh A., Razavi R., Abbasi B., et al. "Modified Alternate-Day Fasting vs. Calorie Restriction in the Treatment of Patients with Metabolic Syndrome: A Randomized Clinical Trial. *Complement Ther Med.* 2019;47:102187.

(13) Lévesque S., Pol J.G., Ferrere G.., Galluzzi L, Zitvogel L., Kroemer G. "Trial Watch: Dietary Interventions for Cancer Therapy." *Oncoimmunology.* 2019;8(7):1591878.

(14) Jockers, D., & Dugan, M. (2020). *The Fasting Transformation: A Functional Guide to Burn Fat, Heal Your Body and Transform Your Life with Intermittent & Extended Fasting.* DrJockers.com.

Appendix

APPENDIX I

What Is Integrative Oncology?

It is unlikely that anyone today has not been affected by cancer in some way, either in themselves or a loved one. Subsequently, many people have learned more about the ways we treat cancer than they ever wanted to know. It is true that over the last 100 years, we have made enormous strides in our knowledge of cancer and how to treat it. From that perspective, there has never been a better time in history to receive a cancer diagnosis. However, cancer is still cancer, and it is a terrifying disease with treatments often equally as horrific. We must do better, and I believe we can.

Conventional oncology (i.e., the treatments used by mainstream cancer centers today) has a strong evidence-based palette of tools to treat cancer. Most people are familiar with these tools, including surgery, chemotherapy, and radiation. Most, however, are less familiar with other standard therapies such as immunotherapy and hormone therapy. Despite these advances, we are still losing the war on cancer—badly. The natural question, then, is: What more can be done? *Can* anything else be done? The answer is a resounding YES! Before we can talk more about what can (and should) be done, it helps to have a brief refresher about the standard treatments currently being used.

Surgery
Surgery involves the physical removal of cancerous tumors from the body. Surgery represents one of the oldest ways in which we have treated cancer, dating to antiquity. Surgery is advised when the cancer is in a location amenable to removal and the patient is physically able to tolerate the procedure. However, surgery is not possible for all types of cancer or for all patients.

Chemotherapy
Chemotherapy involves the use of drugs that have been shown to kill cancer cells. The genesis of chemotherapy occurred when it was observed that people with cancer who were exposed to mustard gas saw remission of their cancer. Chemotherapy has come a long way since that discovery, and it is a useful treatment for almost all types of cancer. Since cancer cells multiply at a much faster rate than healthy cells, they are particularly susceptible to the effects of chemotherapy. As we all know, there are many potential side effects from chemotherapy (as it is typically administered).

Radiation Therapy
Radiation therapy as treatment for cancer reaches back to the early 20th century. This treatment utilizes ionizing radiation to kill cancer and is an effective modality in certain situations. Not surprisingly, there are side effects and a potential for collateral damage from radi-

ation. However, it is important to note that radiation can be much more targeted than it was in the past.

Hormone Therapy

This modality, also referred to as *endocrine therapy*, is utilized to treat cancers which are known to strongly utilize the body's own hormones for energy. In these cases, hormone therapy entails the use of medication to block or decrease the production of specific hormones in the body. As with other treatment modalities, it carries the risk of side effects.

Immunotherapy

Immunotherapy is one of the newest types of cancer treatment to be added to the standard of care and represents a rapidly emerging area of research and discovery. Immunotherapy is essentially harnessing the body's immune system to better recognize and fight cancer.

There is a misconception that a weak immune system is a primary cause of cancer. We must remember that cancer arises from damage to our normal, healthy cells, causing genetic mutations which result in abnormal cellular behavior. The immune system is designed to fight foreign invaders, such as bacteria, viruses, and fungi, which we refer to as "non-self." The immune system is not designed to fight parts of the body recognized as normal, or "self." Thus, cancer is largely able to avoid attack since the immune system cannot typically recognize it as a foreign enemy. In addition, cancer cells have ways to cloak themselves and avoid immune detection.

The work of immunologists such as Dr. James P. Allison and Dr. Tasuku Honjo, which led to their being awarded the Nobel Prize in 2018, has furthered our understanding of immunotherapy significantly. We now know that there are certain proteins on the surfaces of cancer cells that are unique to those cells, differentiating them from normal, healthy cells. Immunotherapy "instructs" the immune system to see these proteins as foreign, giving the body the information it needs to attack cancer cells while ideally leaving normal cells alone.

Immunotherapy is the newest addition to the standard of care, and while it is an exciting area of development, our understanding of it is still rudimentary. The treatments it offers are neither perfect nor void of side effects.

These five therapies combined constitute what is known as the *standard of care* in oncology. These modalities represent the treatments for which we have good evidence of efficacy. Simply put, they work, but they are imperfect.

It is important to remember that these cornerstones of cancer treatment represent some of the most powerful tools we have against cancer. There are decades of research that have yielded reams of evidence supporting their use, and many lives have been saved by employing these therapies.

Many people who find my integrative oncology clinic are interested in modalities beyond the standards of care. Many are searching for treatments to use in lieu of traditional treatments like surgery, chemotherapy, or radiation. Many are disappointed to learn that these treatments are still indicated, even with an integrative approach. It would be shortsighted to dispense with treatments for which we have good evidence, especially against a powerful adversary such as cancer.

This, however, does not mean we do not have significant room for improvement in how we treat cancer. It also does not mean that there are no other treatments available for which good evidence would support their use. There are other great treatments available outside of the standard of care, and this is the fundamental idea behind integrative oncology.

What Is Integrative Oncology?

Integrative oncology is a relatively new approach to how cancer can be treated, and one I hope will eventually become the new normal when it comes to how we treat cancer. Quite simply, integrative oncology combines the best approaches conventional oncology offers with innovative, new techniques from other medical traditions which have shown significant promise. Many of these approaches may not have the level of evidence to be counted as standards of care—yet—but nonetheless have significant evidence supporting their use.

Conventional oncology is often quick to dismiss "alternative" ways of treating cancer, which is understandable. There is a lot of misinformation that exists today about what cancer is and how to treat it. The internet has made such disinformation widely available, and sadly, many people have false ideas about the efficacy of treating cancer "naturally" or via modalities such as diet change or supplementation. In reality, the evidence shows that people who opt to forgo conventional cancer treatment in favor of "natural" remedies have quite poor results. It is no wonder that most oncologists, who spend their days trying to save the lives of people with cancer, simply refuse to take much time to learn anything about alternative cancer treatments.

Conversely, this perspective can be short-sighted as well. The level of evidence necessary for a therapy to be counted among the standard of care is enormous. Studies to "prove" that a therapy works require years of research. This process requires significant funding, with the hope that the treatment under study will prove effective. This, however, does not mean that some treatments that have shown promise—albeit, not the level necessary to be considered standards of care—are *ineffective* or useless. In fact, quite the opposite can be true.

If a treatment shows signs of promise in smaller studies and we believe that it can be safely used without harming the patient, why would we not use every means available to help a patient get better? Particularly when there is good evidence in the literature that certain treatments might have some promise, it seems short-sighted to wait until evidence piles up to the extent that it is approved as part of the standard of care. After all, we are talking about a deadly disease. Using some of these "unproven" therapies as part of a well-rounded integrative oncology approach can potentially save many lives.

In my integrative oncology practice, we include some therapies considered "alternative" or "natural." These include practices such as hypnotherapy, nutrition, supplementation, and stress reduction techniques. It is important to note that these are practices that we use *in tandem* with more evidence-based modalities such as chemotherapy, immunotherapy, and hormone therapy.

While the thrust of this book is to focus on fasting and its many benefits for cancer, it is important to provide a brief introduction to some of the therapies we routinely use in integrative oncology. Many people have likely never heard of integrative oncology, and if so, they might not fully understand what it means.

Treatments in Integrative Oncology

These modalities represent some of what I believe are the most exciting aspects of what we do in my integrative cancer treatment center. Please note that this list of treatments is nowhere near exhaustive. For a more in-depth look at these therapies and others, I recommend reading my bestselling book, *Cancer Secrets*.

Fractionated Chemotherapy

Chemotherapy is perhaps one of the most feared forms of treatment in medicine. Most people are well aware of how unpleasant this treatment can be. Whether you or someone you love has undergone chemotherapy treatment, it is hard not to wonder whether the treatment might be worse than the cancer itself. Undoubtedly, many people likely try to seek more alternative forms of cancer treatment in order to avoid the potential side effects and risks associated with chemotherapy.

Chemotherapy, however, *does* save lives. It remains among the treatments for which we have the best evidence of efficacy in cancer treatment. However, I believe that it can be used in a smarter, safer way. In my practice, we routinely use chemotherapy, but the way we use it differs in several key ways.

Normally, an oncologist calculates the appropriate dosage of chemotherapy based on the current recommended standards. This standard is based on research showing the largest amount of treatment a patient can receive based on his or her specific height and weight. This is what is known as the *maximum tolerated dose*, or *MTD*. This is considered a full-dose treatment of chemotherapy and has been used for many years. As with any treatment, sometimes it works well, but sometimes it does not. Because of this, and because the side effects can be significant, many researchers have called into question the idea that "more is better" when it comes to chemotherapy. (1)

Around twenty years ago, some forward-thinking scientists began testing the use of lower doses of chemotherapy given more frequently. Subsequently, strategies for employing this method of using chemotherapy have been developed. (2, 3) It turns out that there are several benefits to using chemotherapy in this manner.

When patients are given full-dose chemotherapy, you can typically only administer this type of treatment once every one to three weeks, depending on the chemotherapeutic agent(s) involved, the type of cancer, and the stage of the cancer. This is when we see some of the worst side effects associated with chemotherapy, and giving this sort of dosage any more frequently would likely only facilitate even harsher side effects.

However, during that window of time between treatments, the cancer cells that survived the initial treatment have the opportunity to mutate and develop resistance to the chemotherapy agents. We know that tumors contain a percentage of cells highly susceptible to the indicated chemotherapy agents. Large doses of MTD chemotherapy kill these cancer cells but leave many of the resistant cells unaffected, giving them a chance to grow and thrive.

This is one reason we see many cancer patients initially respond positively to full-dose chemotherapy, only to have the cancer fail to continue to respond, or even come back aggressively months or years later. Often, tumors shrink dramatically with the first cycle or two of MTD chemotherapy, but that success is difficult, if not impossible, to maintain once tumors fail to respond to treatments. Remember, chemotherapy only kills the rapidly dividing cancer cells. The cancer cells that aren't undergoing active division—including the notorious cancer stem cells—won't be affected by chemotherapy. Giving a dose only once every few weeks will surely miss many of these more dormant cancer cells.

In my practice, we perform the same dosing calculation a conventional oncologist would to determine the maximum tolerated dosage for a given patient, but we only administer 10–20% of that dosage each treatment. This is what we call *fractionated chemotherapy*. Because the dosage is so much lower, we are able to administer the treatment more frequently, in *metronomic* fashion. Thus, administering lower doses of chemotherapy more often is known as *fractionated metronomic chemotherapy*.

This approach has several key advantages. First, we administer treatment much more often (typically two to three times per week). This means more "hits" to the cancer cells. Because we are administering treatment more often, we stand a greater chance of killing more cancer cells when they are actively growing and dividing (i.e., more susceptible). In addition, administering chemotherapy more often in smaller doses has been shown in research to actually stimulate the immune system, rather than suppress it. Third, the more frequent dosing allows cancer cells less time to develop resistance to the chemotherapy doses being used. Fourth, this approach has been shown to have an anti-angiogenic effect, meaning that cancer is less able to create additional blood supply to itself. (4) Finally, given the lower dosage of chemotherapy, we also see far fewer side effects from treatment, as the collateral damage to healthy cells is greatly mitigated. In other words, the toxicity is typically much lower. (5)

Insulin Potentiation Therapy

Insulin potentiation therapy (IPT) was developed by Dr. Donato

Perez Garcia in Mexico in the 1930s. Dr. Garcia theorized that insulin would improve the cellular uptake of medications, since it was known at the time that insulin was required for the uptake of sugar by cells.

Today, IPT is used by a select group of cancer clinics, including my clinic. We use IPT as a delivery system for chemotherapy, because I believe it allows us to take advantage of some of the metabolic properties associated with cancer. Recall that cancer cells, unlike normal, healthy cells, have a very primitive way of producing energy. Healthy cells go through a multiple-step process that results in the production of over 30 units of ATP (the energy currency of cells). Cancer cells only go through the first step of this process, known as *glycolysis*, wherein glucose (sugar) is metabolized for energy. Because cancer cells rely so heavily on glucose, these cells have a much higher number of insulin receptors on their surface.

With insulin potentiation therapy, we administer insulin in an "off-label" fashion, since insulin's approval by the FDA is to lower blood sugar in diabetics. However, with IPT, the insulin is being used to create a gradient to drive more of whatever is in the blood stream into cancer cells. The goal is to time the insulin with the administration of chemotherapy so that the chemotherapy in the bloodstream is more readily taken up by the cancer cells. We strive to get as much chemotherapy where we need it to go (into the cancer cells) while minimizing its activity elsewhere. In other words, we want to make chemotherapy drugs less like atom bombs and more like heat-seeking missiles.

Many patients say, "Dr. Stegall, administering chemotherapy with IPT makes so much sense! Why isn't this being used in all cancer clinics?" Quite simply, the answer is that insulin potentiation therapy has not undergone a large-scale, long-term clinical trial. While there have been some smaller studies, we simply don't have any significant research on it. The level of research needed to "prove" IPT as an effective delivery system for chemotherapy would take many years and a significant amount of money. Such studies are funded by companies that stand to benefit financially from their monetary investment, and since IPT is a delivery system and not a patentable process, using drugs that have been around for decades, the incentive isn't there. As a result, we will probably never see a large-scale clinical trial on IPT. Without such a trial, it will never be covered by commercial insurance and Medicare, and will thus not become part of the standard of care.

Based on that reality, we are left with a couple of options. The first option is to not use it because it doesn't have the level of evidence we would ideally like to have. That option is certainly understandable, especially for an oncologist who works in a conventional setting and can't deviate from the standard of care in how he treats his patients. The other option is to try IPT and see how it works. That was the decision I made, after seeing the effects of the maximum tolerated dose given in the conventional fashion in many patients I cared for. Because I have my own practice, I was able to incorporate IPT with my patients and see for myself how it works. I'm glad I did, because I have seen it be a very effective and safe method of administering chemotherapy.

Despite the lack of large-scale clinical trials, we do have some studies that illuminate how IPT functions. It is believed that IPT affects the metabolism of cancer cells, making them more susceptible to chemotherapy. Subsequently, this allows us to simultaneously use a lower dose of chemotherapy drugs—but with greater efficacy. Insulin given with chemotherapy better targets the drugs to cancer cells.

(6) This is consistent with research that confirms cancer cells have a greater number of insulin and glucose receptors on their surfaces than normal, healthy cells.

Lymphatic Drainage Therapy

Lymph drainage was a term first coined by Canadian physician Dr. Frederic Millard in the 1920s, but the process was largely developed in the 1930s by Drs. Emil and Estrid Vodder. (7, 8) The process was perfected by French physician Dr. Bruno Chikly, who formed the basis of the kind of lymphatic drainage therapy we employ today. (9) Dr. Chikly was the first to point out the benefits associated with this type of therapy, including stimulation of the immune system, elimination of toxins, enhancement of the nervous system, and improved circulation of various body fluids including lymph, interstitial fluid, cerebrospinal fluid, and blood.

The lymphatic system serves some very important purposes in the body. Among the most important of its roles is that the lymphatic system is essentially the training ground for our immune system. The lymphatic system runs parallel to the bloodstream; when the bone marrow makes white blood cells, these cells are ushered into the lymphatic system. It is here that white blood cells learn how to protect the body against pathogens. After receiving training in the lymphatic system, white blood cells are flooded into the bloodstream, where they serve the purpose of fighting any foreign invaders, keeping us safe from infection.

Often with cancer patients, there is some level of lymphatic involvement, particularly when cancers have spread to the lymph nodes. Invariably, the surgical removal of lymph nodes results in congestion within the lymphatic system, which reduces the flow of lymph, resulting in some level of immune system disruption. An extreme example of lymph congestion can be seen in lymphedema, which often results in a significantly swollen arm on the side of mastectomy and lymph node removal in women who have undergone mastectomy.

Lymph nodes exist throughout the body, but they exist in higher concentrations in the neck, armpit, and groin. A skilled lymph drainage therapist can determine where congestion exists in the lymphatic system. Once those areas are identified, we can break up the congested fluid using non-invasive equipment designed specifically to promote better lymph flow.

We have had incredible results using lymphatic drainage therapy in my practice. Some have come into the office unable to lift their arms above horizontal due to lymphedema. After only a couple weeks of regular treatment, much of their mobility returned. In addition to assisting with lymphedema, I believe lymph drainage therapy plays an important role in helping the body fight cancer and detoxify. This is especially true in patients who have a significant burden of lymph node involvement from cancer. The lymphatic drainage therapy treatment sessions are not only helpful from a therapeutic standpoint, but are also quite relaxing for patients.

Repurposed Medications

Many drugs that have been developed, rigorously tested, and approved to treat non-cancerous conditions have been found in subsequent research to also have anticancer activity. When a drug is used for a purpose other than what it was initially developed and approved for, this is known as *off-label use*.

The off-label use of pharmaceuticals by physicians is considered acceptable when there is scientific evidence that the drug might help, coupled with a low likelihood of harm. One of the benefits of repurposing medication to better fight cancer is that we already understand how safely they can be used, at what doses they may be used, and any contraindications for using these drugs, because they all have been through the rigorous testing of large-scale clinical trials and subsequently deemed safe. Since we know that these medications can be used safely and believe that they might help fight cancer in a unique way, why would we *not* use them as part of our anti-cancer regimen?

Unfortunately, this idea has not become part of the mainstream practice of oncology. I believe this is considerably short-sighted, considering the fact that we are still badly losing the war on cancer. As long as these drugs are used in a clinical setting under the supervision of a qualified physician who has experience with their use, there is seemingly little reason to not use them.

A research paper published in 2012 entitled "Hiding in Plain Sight" sought to determine whether many existing pharmaceuticals possessed any sort of anti-cancer effect. This paper highlighted many exciting candidates, but importantly the researchers stated, "We advocate that confirmation of these findings in randomized trials be considered a high research priority, as the potential impact on human lives saved could be immense." (10) This is the paradigm we embrace in my clinic, and hopefully it will one day become the new normal in oncology.

I have included some notable examples here of medications that can be repurposed to help fight cancer. This is not an exhaustive list by any means but is used here for illustrative purposes. A properly crafted protocol of repurposed medications takes time, with careful consideration required to ensure that the medications chosen are safe for each patient with regard for the other medications, supplements, and treatments the patient is receiving. Remember, many of these are prescription medications, so this is not a do-it-yourself endeavor. Please consult a physician who has experience with these medications in the cancer setting, as there are many nuances here that must be considered.

Aspirin

Acetylsalicylic acid (ASA), commonly known as aspirin, is derived from the bark of the willow tree. We have known for a while that people who take aspirin lower their risk of developing cancer, especially colorectal cancer. One study showed that taking a daily aspirin resulted in a 24% reduction in risk for developing colorectal cancer. The benefit was apparent after five years of daily use. (11)

Aspirin may also be beneficial for those already diagnosed with cancer; another study evaluated the use of low-dose aspirin in cancer treatment and found it could increase survival by 20% and reduce metastasis. (12)

The use of aspirin should be monitored by your oncologist, because it is a blood thinner and can interact with other medications. However, for the majority of patients, it is well-tolerated, easy to incorporate, and subsequently a good candidate for inclusion in an anti-cancer protocol.

Cimetidine

Cimetidine is commonly used to treat gastroesophageal reflux disease (GERD) and peptic ulcers. Cimetidine blocks the histamine receptor known as H2. Cimetidine has shown anti-tumor activity in the treatment of colorectal cancer, (13) kidney cancer, (14) and melanoma. (15) Studies indicate that cimetidine helps maintain lymphocyte counts and natural killer (NK) cell counts, both of which are important markers of immune system activity. (16)

Cimetidine can inhibit the action of other drugs, so its use must be monitored.

Clarithromycin (Biaxin)
Clarithromycin is a part of the class of antibiotics known as *macrolide antibiotics*. It is used to treat infections, specifically in the sinuses, lungs, and gastrointestinal tract. It is also used to treat Lyme disease. Clarithromycin has shown a few notable anti-cancer properties. It inhibits nuclear factor kappa beta (NF-kB) and suppresses tumor necrosis factor alpha (TNF-alpha). It is also thought to prevent angiogenesis, which, again, is vital to suppressing cancer's ability to supply itself with nutrients. (17) Finally, clarithromycin has been shown to reduce cachexia, which is the wasting syndrome typically seen in advanced cancers which causes loss of appetite, fatigue, weight loss, and muscle atrophy.

In one study of 49 patients with inoperable lung cancer, those who received clarithromycin survived twice as long on average compared to those who did not receive the drug. (18)

Dipyridamole
Dipyridamole is a drug used to reduce the activity of platelets, which are a necessary component of blood clotting. It is commonly used for preventing blood clots in patients prone to heart attacks and strokes.

Elevated platelets are often seen in cancer patients, which is one reason cancer patients tend to have more blood clots than non-cancer patients. Elevated platelets also point toward the presence of inflammation; the downstream effect of these elevated platelets and inflammation is the recruitment of growth factors, which facilitates the spread of cancer. Thus, blocking platelets can have a powerful anti-cancer effect, and in this regard, there have been some promising studies involving dipyridamole.

One particularly notable study looked at pancreatic cancer patients who received dipyridamole along with the standard of care regimen. These patients had poor prognoses because none of them were surgical candidates; this put their predicted survival to be between 8 and 12 months. In the 38 patients studied, 70% survived one year and 27% were ultimately able to undergo surgery to remove the cancer. These patients had a one-year survival rate of 83%, far superior to the conventional standard, which was attributed to dipyridamole. (19)

Disulfiram (Antabuse)

Disulfiram was developed in the 1920s to treat alcoholism. When taken, disulfiram inhibits enzymes in the liver that help break down alcohol, resulting in severe hangover symptoms. It was popular for a time, but fell out of favor as newer drugs were developed.

Disulfiram, however, has significant anti-cancer activity. It directly causes apoptosis (cell death) of many different cancer cells. It inhibits a component of cancer cells known as *nuclear factor kappa beta* (*NF-kB*), a pathway that controls cancer growth and development. Studies indicate that disulfiram has anti-tumor, anti-metastatic, and anti-angiogenic properties, all at non-toxic doses. (20)

Not surprisingly, alcohol must be entirely avoided while taking disulfiram, even in the tiniest doses seen in some herbal tinctures.

Itraconazole

Itraconazole is a broad-spectrum anti-fungal drug shown to have an anti-cancer effect. There are some interesting similarities between fungi and cancer. Both thrive on sugar as an energy source, both produce ATP in the absence of oxygen, and both accumulate lactic acid. There are numerous studies confirming that fungi, and their secondary byproducts, known as mycotoxins, can cause DNA damage that leads to cancer. (21, 22)

Itraconazole showed modest anti-cancer activity in men with advanced prostate cancer. (23) Other studies have also been encouraging. Itraconazole should be taken with a good probiotic supplement, as it can damage beneficial gut bacteria. This internal flora consisting of "good" bacteria is responsible for many health benefits, including aiding in digestion, manufacturing certain nutrients, and assisting in immunity.

Mebendazole

This anti-parasitic medication is approved to treat pinworms, roundworms, and hookworms, but it also has documented anticancer effects. Studies have shown that mebendazole inhibits a pathway known as *matrix metalloproteinase-2* (*MMP-2*), critical for cancer growth. It also addresses abnormal communication networks between cancer cells by inhibiting the Hedgehog pathway.

In addition, and perhaps most importantly, mebendazole disrupts microtubules, which are key to cancer cell division. This is a similar mechanism by which chemotherapy drugs such as paclitaxel and vincristine operate.

Finally, research indicates that mebendazole is synergistic with a wide range of other medications, including chemotherapy. (24)

Metformin

This drug is used as a first-line treatment in type 2 diabetics for controlling blood sugar. Interestingly, researchers have noted that diabetics taking metformin had a 54% lower risk of developing cancer than diabetics not taking metformin. (25)

There are several mechanisms by which metformin has an anti-cancer effect. The most prominent is the inhibition of the mammalian target of rapamycin (mTOR) pathway. (26) The mTOR pathway is a major factor in cancer cell growth, spread, and survival. (27) If we can inhibit this pathway, we enhance our ability to slow down cancer growth and metastasis.

Metformin is also thought to elicit an anti-cancer effect by reducing insulin and insulin-like growth factor 1(IGF-1), which are both heavily utilized by cancer cells. (28)

Metformin has also been shown to kill cancer stem cells. You can think of cancer stem cells as dormant cells which are not actively dividing (and thus not harmed by chemotherapy), which can become "activated" and eventually result in the spread of cancer. Metformin's ability to kill these cancer stem cells makes it an important tool for preventing and treating cancer.

Metformin is very safe, and side effects (when they occur) are typically mild and transient. These can often be avoided by using an extended-release form of the medication.

Naltrexone

Naltrexone was developed in the 1980s to assist patients in overcoming drug addiction. It works by blocking the opioid receptor, reducing the addiction potential of opiate drugs. A secondary effect of blocking the opioid receptor, however, is the inhibition of beta-endorphin and metenkephalin. Inhibiting these two factors has the effect of boosting the immune system. The anti-cancer benefit seems to be derived from the increase in both the number and activity of natural killer cells that are the result of the immune-boosting effects of naltrexone. (29) Natural killer cells are an important part of the immune system and are often deficient in cancer patients.

We have learned that we can achieve these powerful, immune-modulating effects by using very low doses of naltrexone, approximately 10% of what would be used in treating addiction. Naltrexone is inexpensive, but must be made by a compounding pharmacist in the lower doses we require. It is very safe, and the only known side effect is vivid dreams.

Propranolol

Propranolol is in a class of antihypertensive medications known as *beta-blockers*. These drugs act against beta-adrenergic receptors. Beta-adrenergic receptors are part of the sympathetic nervous system, which governs our body's fight-or-flight response. Beta-blockers lower blood pressure by blocking these receptors.

Propranolol—along with other beta-blockers—has also been shown to possess anti-cancer effects. Epidemiological studies on men taking beta-blockers for high blood pressure reveal that those taking beta-blockers in lieu of other blood pressure medication had a lower risk of developing prostate cancer. (30) Another study showed that cancer patients taking a beta-blocker had a lower risk of dying from cancer. (31)

Importantly, the fact that beta-blockers work against cancer highlights an important and often overlooked component of cancer: the role that stress plays in cancer. Because beta-blockers work by reducing the fight-or-flight portion of the nervous system, the stress—or perceived stress—on the body is reduced significantly. One recent study confirmed that stress-induced activation of the neuroendocrine system resulted in a 30-fold increase in cancer spread. (32)

In my practice, stress reduction is a very important part of our integrative cancer treatment protocols. We emphasize stress identification as well as stress reduction, and begin this emphasis on the first day of treatment with all patients. This is not just important for cancer patients, however. We all have stress in our lives, and there are more chronic and acute stressors in modern society than ever before. Daily stress reduction practices such as prayer, meditation, laughter, and spending time with those we love are not only crucial to happiness, but also to overall health and the prevention and treatment of cancer.

Rapamycin

Rapamycin is a natural substance produced by the bacteria *Streptomyces hygroscopicus*. It was first isolated on Easter Island in the southeastern Pacific Ocean in the 1970s, and it is the only known place on Earth it has been found. Rapamycin was used initially as an anti-fungal compound because it targets a component of yeast cells known as *target of rapamycin*, or TOR. Later, it was found that rapamycin suppressed the immune system in humans, as TOR is also found in mammalian cells. In humans, this target is known as mTOR, which stands for *mammalian target of rapamycin* (sometimes referred to as *mechanistic target of rapamycin*). (33) We know that mTOR is responsible for many key cellular functions, such as growth and energy production. It can be thought of as a gas pedal that causes the cell to "go." It is a necessary component of healthy cells, but also something we want to limit, as it has been shown in studies to contribute to aging and decreased lifespan.

Almost always, mTor is hijacked by cancer cells, and rapamycin can be used to block this pathway. This is partly responsible for the aggressive growth we see in cancer cells. Rapamycin suppresses this mTor pathway, but we must be careful, because too much rapamycin suppresses the immune system. Not surprisingly, rapamycin is approved to prevent rejection after organ transplantation. Thus, the dose is critical.

For anticancer purposes, rapamycin is used in lower doses. In addition, rather than taking it daily as is customary for organ transplant patients, we dose it intermittently (in "pulsatile" fashion). This approach is quite effective in blocking mTor, while avoiding the immunosuppressive effects. In fact, rapamycin is now considered a longevity drug due to its ability to extend lifespan in yeast, flies, and mice. (34)

Statins

You might be aware that statins are prescribed to lower cholesterol. In recent years, they have come under scrutiny for their side effects, including the fact that they increase the risk of developing type 2 diabetes. From a cardiovascular perspective, I believe they are overprescribed. However, statins might have a lot to offer with regard to cancer.

Statins have several beneficial effects when it comes to fighting cancer, including reduced inflammation, enhancement of the immune system, and anti-angiogenic effects. Unsurprisingly, studies show they have beneficial cancer-preventative effects. One study found that people taking statins have a 47% reduction in risk for developing colorectal cancer. (35) Another study found that patients taking statins for at least six months had a 55% reduction in risk for developing lung cancer. (36) Another study noted that statins might reduce the risk of developing prostate cancer. (37)

Statins may also have benefits for those already diagnosed with cancer. One study of liver cancer patients who were not candidates for surgery noted that those who took statins lived twice as long as those who did not. (38) Another study found that in men who had prostate cancer and had their prostates surgically removed, those who took a statin had a 30% lower chance of having cancer recurrence. Those who took the highest doses of statins had even better results, which was a 50% lower chance of recurrence. (39)

The decision to use statins in cancer treatment must be considered carefully. The anti-cancer effect of statins is likely due to their ability to reduce inflammation and inhibit angiogenesis. However, statins do reduce cholesterol, which may not necessarily be a good thing. Cholesterol is a necessary component of cell membranes and the production of hormones. Thus, thorough testing, including a lipid panel to measure total cholesterol, LDL cholesterol, HDL cholesterol, and triglycerides, is an important first step to assessing a patient's candidacy for statin use.

As mentioned earlier, this is not an exhaustive list of medications we use in repurposed fashion to treat cancer. However, it should be clear that these medications, which are typically safe and have been around for decades, provide an excellent illustration of our need to think outside the box when it comes to cancer and how we treat it. There are many more treatments and therapies I consider valid and useful when it comes to cancer, and each of these has a very specific role to play. Some examples include sonophotodynamic therapy, hyperthermia, mind-body therapy, pulsed electromagnetic field therapy, and certainly various nutritional supplements.

References

(1) Fidler I.J. and Ellis L.M. "Chemotherapeutic Drugs - More Really Is Not Better." *Nat Med* 2000;6(5):500-02.

(2) Hanahan D., Bergers G., Bergsland E. "Less Is More, Regularly: Metronomic Dosing of Cytotoxic Drugs Can Target Tumor Angiogenesis in Mice." *J Clin Invest* 2000;105:1045-47.

(3) Kareva I., Waxman D.J., and Klement G.L. "Metronomic Chemotherapy: An Attractive Alternative to Maximum Tolerated Dose Therapy That Can Activate Anti-Tumor Immunity and Minimize Therapeutic Resistance." *Cancer Lett* 2015 Mar 28; 358(2): 100-106.

(4) Browder T., Butterfield C.E., Kraling B.M., et al. "Antiangiogenic Scheduling of Chemotherapy Improves Efficacy against Experimental Drug-Resistant Cancer." *Cancer Res* 2000;60(7):1878-86.

(5) Klement G., Baruchel S., Ran J., et al. "Continuous Low-Dose Therapy with Vinblastine and VEGF Receptor-2 Antibody Induces Sustained Tumor Regression without Overt Toxicity." *J Clin Invest* 2000;105(8):R15-24.

(6) Ayre S.G., Garcia y Bellon D.P., Garcia D.P. Jr. "Insulin, Chemotherapy, and the Mechanisms of Malignancy: The Design and Demise of Cancer." *Med Hypotheses* 2000;55(4):330-34.

(7) Millard F.P. "Applied Anatomy of the Lymphatics." Kirksville: International Lymphatic Research Society, 1922.

(8) French, RM. *The Complete Guide to Lymph Drainage Massage*, Clifton Park: Milady, 2011.

(9) Chikly, Bruno. "Lymph Drainage Therapy and Its Integration in a Massage Therapy Practice." *American Massage Therapy Association*, page 20. URL http://www.iahe.com/images/pdf/3319_001.pdf.

(10) Holmes, Michelle D., and Wendy Y Chen. "Hiding in Plain View: The Potential for Commonly Used Drugs to Reduce Breast Cancer Mortality." *Breast Cancer Research*, vol. 14, no. 2, 2012, doi:10.1186/bcr3336.

(11) Garcia-Albeniz X., Chan A.T. "Aspirin for the Prevention of Colorectal Cancer." *Best Practices Res Clin Gastroenterol* 2011;25(0):461-72.

(12) Elwood P.C., Morgan G., Pickering J.E., et al. "Aspirin in the Treatment of Cancer: Reductions in Metastatic Spread and in Mortality: A Systematic Review and Meta-Analyses of Published Studies." *PLoS One* 2016;11(4):e0152402.

(13) Adams W.J., Morris D.L. "Short-Course Cimetidine and Survival with Colorectal Cancer." *Lancet* 1994; 344: 8939-8940.

(14) Nagano T., Matsuda H., Park Y.C., et al. "Successful Treatment of Metastatic Renal Cell Carcinoma with Cimetidine - Report of Two Cases." *Nihon Hinyokika Gakkai Zasshi* 1996;87(10):1201-04.

(15) Borgstrom S., et al. "Human Leukocyte Interferon and Cimetidine for Metastatic Melanoma." *N Engl J Med* 1982; 307(17): 1080-1081.

(16) Katoh J., et al. "Cimetidine Reduces Impairment of Cellular Immunity after Cardiac Operations with Cardiopulmonary Bypass." *J Thorac Cardiovasc Surg* 1998; 116(2): 312-318.

(17) Yatsunami J., Fukuno Y., Nagata M., et al. "Anti-Angiogenic and Anti-Tumor Effects of 14-Membered Ring Macrolides on Mouse B16 Melanoma Cells." *Clin Exp Metastasis* 1999;17(4):361-67.

(18) Mikasa K., Sawaki M., Kita E., et al. "Significant Survival Benefit to Patients with Advanced Non-Small-Cell Lung Cancer from Treatment with Clarithromycin." *Chemotherapy* 1997;43(4):288-96.

(19) Todd K.E., Gloor B., Lane J.S., et al. "Resection of Locally Advanced Pancreatic Cancer after Down Staging with Continuous-Infusion 5-Fluoruracil, Mitomycin-C, Leucovorin, and Dipyridamole." *J Gastrointest Surg* 1998;2(2):159-66.

(20) Sauna Z.E., Shukla S., and Ambudkar S.V. "Disulfiram, an Old Drug with New Potential Therapeutic Uses for Human Cancers and Fungal Infections." *Mol BioSyst* 2005;1:127-34.

(21) Wang J.S. and Groopman J. "DNA Damage by Mycotoxins." *Mutation Research* 1999;424:167-81.

(22) Liu Y. and Wu F. "Global Burden of Aflatoxin-Induced Hepatocellular Carcinoma: A Risk Assessment." *Environmental Health Perspectives* 2010;118:818-24.

(23) Antonarakis E.S., Heath E.L., Smith D.C., et al. "Repurposing Itraconazole as a Treatment for Advanced Prostate Cancer: A Noncooperative Randomized Phase II Trial in Men with Metastatic Castration-Resistant Prostate Cancer." *Oncologist* 2013; 18(2):163-173.

(24) Guerini A.E., Triggiani L., Maddalo M., et al. "Mebendazole as a Candidate for Drug Repurposing in Oncology: An Extensive Review of Current Literature." *Cancers (Basel)* 2019; 11(9): 1284. doi: 10.3390/cancers11091284

(25) Libby G., Donnelly L.A., Donnan P.T., et al. "New Users of Metformin Are at Low Risk of Incident Cancer: A Cohort Study Among People with Type 2 Diabetes." *Diabetes Care* 2009 Sep; 32(9): 1620-1625.

(26) Chiang G.G., Abraham R.T. "Targeting the mTOR Signaling Network in Cancer." *Trends Mol Med* 2007; 13: 433-442.

(27) Guertin D.A., Sabatini D.M. "Defining the Role of mTOR in Cancer." *Cancer Cell* 2007 Jul; 12(1): 9-22.

(28) LeRoith D., Roberts C.T. "Insulin-Like Growth Factors and Cancer." *Ann Intern Med* 1995; 122: 54-59.

(29) Mathews P.M., Froelich C.J., Sibbitt W.L., et al. "Enhancement of Natural Cytotoxicity by Beta-Endorphin." *J Immune* 1983;130(4):1658-62.

(30) Perron L., Bairati I., Harel F., et al. "Antihypertensive Drug Use and the Risk of Prostate Cancer" (Canada). *Cancer Causes Control* 2004;15(6):535-41.

(31) Zhong S., Yu D., Zhang X., et al. "B-Blocker Use and Mortality in Cancer Patients: Systematic Review and Meta-Analysis of Observational Studies." *Eur J Cancer Prev* 2016;25(5):440-48.

(32) Sloan E.K., Priceman S.J., Cox B.F., et al. "The Sympathetic Nervous System Induces a Metastatic Switch in Primary Breast Cancer." *Cancer Res* 2010;70(18):7042-52.

(33) Dumont F.J. and Su Q. "Mechanism of Action of the Immunosuppressant Rapamycin." *Life Sci* 1996;58(5):373-95.

(34) Blagosklonny M. "Rapamycin for Longevity: Opinion Article." *Aging* (Albany NY) 2019; 11(19): 8048-67. doi: 10.18632/aging.102355.

(35) Poynter J.N., Gruber S.B., Higgins P.D.R., et al. "Statins and the Risk of Colorectal Cancer." *N Engl J Med* 2005;352:2184-92.

(36) Khurana V., Bejjanki H.R., Caldito G., et al. "Statins Reduce the Risk of Lung Cancer in Humans: A Large Case-Control Study o US Veterans." *Chest* 2007;131(5):1282-88.

(37) Bansal D., Undela K., D'Cruz S., et al. "Statin Use and Risk of Prostate Cancer: A Meta-Analysis of Observational Studies." *PLoS One* 2012;7(10):e46691.

(38) Kawata S., Yamasaki E., Nagase T., et al. "Effect of Pravastatin on Survival in Patients with Advanced Hepatocellular Carcinoma. A Randomized Clinical Trial." *Br J Cancer* 2001;84(7):886-91.

(39) Hamilton R.J., Banez L.L., Aronson W.J., et al. "Statin Medication Use and the Risk of Biochemical Recurrence after Radical Prostatectomy." *Cancer* 2010;116(14):3389-98.

Printed in Dunstable, United Kingdom